MW01181711

ANTI

INFLAMMATORY

DIET

YOUR ALLY FOR

HEALTH

Unveils the secret to halting inflammation, bolstering the immune system, and energizing metabolism for a rejuvenated body.

by

Giuliano Monti

Summary

Chapter 1: Introduction to Inflammation

1.1 Definition and Role of Inflammation in the Body

Inflammation is a fundamental biological process that plays a crucial role in our body's immune system. It's a natural and protective response to infections, injuries, or diseases, aiming to eliminate the cause of irritation and initiate the healing process. To understand the importance of an anti-inflammatory diet, it's essential to start with a thorough understanding of inflammation and its impact on the human body.

When tissue damage occurs, such as a wound or infection, the body reacts by releasing chemicals that trigger an inflammatory response. This response includes increased blood flow to the affected area, the release of antibodies and proteins, as well as the arrival of immune system cells to fight off invaders. This process is critical for healing and is usually observed through symptoms like redness, warmth, swelling, and pain.

Although inflammation is an essential part of the body's immune response, it's not always beneficial. When inflammation becomes chronic, it can have harmful effects and contribute to the development of several chronic diseases. Chronic inflammation occurs when the body's inflammatory response doesn't stop as it should. Instead, it continues to persist, causing progressive damage to tissues. This type of inflammation is subtle and often doesn't show immediate symptoms, but over time it can lead to diseases such as arthritis, heart disease, diabetes, and even some types of cancer.

One of the main causes of chronic inflammation is lifestyle, particularly diet. Foods that exacerbate inflammation include those high in refined sugars, saturated fats, and trans fats. These foods can alter the balance of chemicals in the body, promoting chronic inflammatory processes. Conversely, a diet rich in anti-inflammatory foods, such as fresh fruits and vegetables, healthy fats, and lean proteins, can help reduce inflammation and promote overall health.

The aim of this book, therefore, is to provide a comprehensive guide to adopting an anti-inflammatory dietary regimen. Starting with an in-depth understanding of inflammation and its impact on health, we can explore how specific changes in diet and lifestyle can help manage, reduce, and even prevent chronic inflammation. This approach will not only contribute to improving overall health but will also offer a solid foundation for lasting well-being.

As we progress through the book, we will explore in more detail the links between specific foods and inflammation, providing practical information and advice on how to adopt an effective anti-inflammatory diet. With this knowledge, you will be able to make informed decisions about your diet and lifestyle, setting you on a path to health and wellness.

1.2 Difference Between Acute and Chronic Inflammation

After introducing the concept of inflammation in the previous section, it's important to distinguish between the two main types of inflammation: acute and chronic. This distinction is crucial for understanding how inflammation affects our health and how we can modify its impact through diet and lifestyle.

Acute Inflammation: The Immediate Protective Response

Acute inflammation is the body's rapid, short-term response to physical damage, an infection, or another immediate challenge. It is characterized by well-known symptoms such as redness, warmth, swelling, and pain. These signs indicate that the immune system is working to fight off infection, remove harmful stimuli, and initiate the healing process. For example, if you cut your finger or have a bacterial infection, acute inflammation helps to isolate the area and fight pathogens.

Acute inflammation is essential for our survival. Without it, relatively minor injuries or common infections could be fatal. This type of inflammation usually resolves quickly, leaving the body in its original state of health without long-term effects.

Chronic Inflammation: A Silent Threat

Unlike acute inflammation, chronic inflammation is a slow, prolonged process that can last for months or years. Instead of aiding in healing, chronic inflammation can damage the body's cells and alter the normal functions of organs. This type of inflammation often lacks immediate symptoms, making it insidious and dangerous.

Chronic inflammation is associated with numerous long-term diseases, including arthritis, heart disease, type 2 diabetes, obesity, autoimmune diseases, and certain types of cancer. Factors such as a poor diet, lack of physical activity, smoking, obesity, pollution, and chronic stress can contribute to chronic inflammation.

The Link Between the Two Types of Inflammation

While acute inflammation is a necessary and beneficial response, chronic inflammation represents a dysfunction of the immune system. The transition from acute to chronic inflammation can occur when the body is exposed to continuous inflammatory stimuli or when the inflammatory process fails to resolve completely.

Understanding the difference between these two types of inflammation is crucial for developing prevention and treatment strategies. Through diet and lifestyle choices, we can influence our immune system and reduce the risk of chronic inflammation.

In the next section, we will explore how chronic inflammation can contribute to the development of many chronic diseases. This will allow us to better understand why adopting a proactive approach to reduce inflammation through diet and lifestyle is so important. This understanding will form the basis for the practical recommendations and dietary changes that will be discussed in the following chapters.

1.3 Impact of Chronic Inflammation on Health

After exploring the difference between acute and chronic inflammation, it's crucial to understand how the latter impacts our health. Chronic inflammation is a common underlying factor in many long-term diseases. This section focuses on the impact of chronic inflammation and lays the groundwork for understanding the importance of combating it through diet and lifestyle.

The Central Role in Disease Etiology

Chronic inflammation has been identified as a primary cause of many chronic diseases. This form of inflammation acts slowly and insidiously, damaging body tissues over time. Diseases such as rheumatoid arthritis, cardiovascular diseases, type 2 diabetes, obesity, certain forms of cancer, and neurodegenerative diseases like Alzheimer's are strongly linked to chronic inflammation.

Pathological Mechanisms

In conditions of chronic inflammation, the immune system continues to release inflammatory cells even in the absence of infections or injuries. These cells can end up attacking healthy tissues, causing progressive damage and a series of reactions that further perpetuate inflammation. Over time, this process can lead to cellular function alteration and tissue degeneration.

Inflammation and Cardiovascular Diseases

One of the most studied connections is between chronic inflammation and cardiovascular diseases. Inflammation can contribute to the buildup of plaques in arteries (atherosclerosis), increasing the risk of heart attack and stroke. Risk factors such as a diet high in saturated fats, smoking, and lack of exercise can exacerbate this process.

Inflammation and Metabolism

Metabolism is also affected by chronic inflammation. Conditions like obesity can lead to a form of low-grade inflammation, which in turn contributes to the development of type 2 diabetes. This vicious circle between inflammation, weight gain, and insulin resistance underscores the importance of a healthy diet and lifestyle.

Connecting the Dots Between Inflammation and Diet

The link between chronic inflammation and various diseases underscores the importance of preventive strategies. One of the most effective weapons against chronic inflammation is a well-balanced diet rich in anti-inflammatory foods. In the next section, we will examine the factors contributing to chronic inflammation, focusing particularly on how certain lifestyles and dietary habits can fuel it. This will allow us to establish a clear connection between daily choices and their influence on chronic inflammation, setting the stage for introducing specific dietary changes in the following chapters.

1.4 Factors Contributing to Chronic Inflammation

Having understood the significant impact of chronic inflammation on health, it's now essential to examine the factors that contribute to this condition. Understanding these causes is the first step towards mitigating their effects and laying the groundwork for effective changes in lifestyle and diet, as will be discussed in the following sections and chapters.

Diet and Inflammation

One of the primary contributors to chronic inflammation is diet. Foods high in refined sugars, saturated fats, and trans fats can trigger inflammatory processes in the body. Conversely, a diet lacking in fresh fruits and vegetables limits the intake of antioxidants and essential nutrients that fight inflammation. Developing anti-inflammatory meal plans, which will be addressed in later chapters, aims to reduce the intake of these pro-inflammatory foods and increase the intake of anti-inflammatory ones.

Sedentary Lifestyle

A lack of physical activity is another significant factor. A sedentary lifestyle can contribute to weight gain and obesity, which are closely linked to chronic inflammation. Regular physical exercise, on the other hand, not only helps maintain a healthy weight but also produces direct anti-inflammatory effects.

Smoking and Alcohol

Cigarette smoking and excessive alcohol consumption are two habits that significantly exacerbate inflammation. Smoking contributes to chronic inflammation and increases the risk of developing inflammation-related diseases. Similarly, excessive alcohol can cause inflammation and damage organs such as the liver.

Stress and Mental Health

Chronic stress, both physical and psychological, is a powerful trigger of inflammation. The prolonged response to stress can lead to a continuous release of inflammatory hormones. Therefore, stress management plays a crucial role in reducing inflammation, a theme that will be further explored in later chapters.

Environmental Factors

Finally, environmental factors such as exposure to pollutants, toxic chemicals, and allergens can contribute to chronic inflammation. While we cannot always fully control our environment, becoming aware of these factors can help reduce exposure.

In summary, chronic inflammation is influenced by a variety of factors, many of which are under our direct or indirect control. By modifying our diet, increasing physical activity, quitting excessive smoking and alcohol, managing stress, and reducing exposure to harmful environmental factors, we can significantly lower the risk of chronic inflammation.

The next section, 1.5, will bridge the overview of factors contributing to chronic inflammation with an overview of the book, outlining the objectives and structure of the text, and preparing the reader to fully dive into the chapters that follow, where these insights will be turned into concrete actions.

1.5 Book Overview and Objectives

After outlining the importance of inflammation and its effects on health, as well as the factors contributing to chronic inflammation, it's time to delve deeper into the structure and objectives of this book. This overview serves to prepare the reader for the journey ahead, setting expectations and outlining the path we will take together.

Book Structure

The book is divided into ten chapters, each dedicated to a specific aspect of the anti-inflammatory diet and its impact on health. The initial chapters provide a theoretical foundation, exploring inflammation and its connection with diet and lifestyle. Subsequent chapters focus on practical advice and specifics, including detailed meal plans, tips for diet modification, and the incorporation of physical exercises and stress management techniques. The goal is to offer a comprehensive guide that not only informs but also provides the necessary tools for making real and lasting changes.

Book Objectives

The primary objective of this book is to equip the reader with the knowledge and resources to adopt an anti-inflammatory lifestyle. The goals include:

- Education: Providing detailed information on inflammation and its impact on health.

- Prevention: Demonstrating how an anti-inflammatory diet can prevent or reduce chronic inflammation and related diseases.

- Practical action: Offering meal plans and practical advice for adopting an anti-inflammatory diet.

- Holistic support: Integrating dietary changes with advice on physical exercise, stress management, and other lifestyle aspects.

- Motivation: Inspiring the reader to undertake and maintain these changes, showing the long-term benefits of an anti-inflammatory lifestyle.

Importance of Consistency and Continuity

Throughout each chapter, themes and information are presented consistently and logically, ensuring that each section effectively connects to the next. This consistency helps build a gradual and profound understanding of the subject, allowing the reader to easily integrate the information into their life.

Transition to the Next Section

Concluding this introductory chapter, the reader now possesses a solid understanding of inflammation and its contributing factors. In the next section, we will begin to explore more closely the direct link between diet and inflammation. Chapter 2 will open with an in-depth discussion on how certain foods can exacerbate or mitigate chronic inflammation, thus laying the groundwork for the informed dietary choices we will explore throughout the rest of the book.

Chapter 2: Diet and Inflammation

2.1 Correlation Between Diet and Inflammation

Beginning the second chapter, we will explore the fundamental link between diet and inflammation. This section lays the groundwork for understanding how specific foods and dietary patterns influence inflammation in the body, preparing the reader for a more detailed analysis of specific foods in the following sections.

The Power of Foods in Modulating Inflammation

Diet plays a crucial role in modulating inflammation. Certain foods can trigger inflammatory processes, while others can act as powerful anti-inflammatory agents. This effect is due to the variety of nutrients, antioxidants, and bioactive compounds present in foods, which interact with the body's biological pathways. For instance, foods rich in omega-3 fatty acids, such as fatty fish, can reduce inflammation, whereas those high in saturated fats and refined sugars can promote it.

The Role of Diet in Inflammatory Onset

Scientific studies have shown that high-glycemic diets, rich in processed foods and lacking in essential nutrients, are associated with higher levels of inflammatory markers in the blood. These markers, such as C-reactive protein (CRP), are reliable indicators of systemic inflammation and are often elevated in conditions like obesity, metabolic syndrome, and type 2 diabetes.

The Role of Gut Microbiota

A less known, yet equally important, aspect is the impact of diet on the gut microbiota. The microbiota, composed of billions of bacteria residing in our intestines, plays a vital role in regulating inflammation. A diet rich in fiber, prebiotics, and probiotics can promote a healthy microbiota, which in turn can help reduce systemic inflammation. Conversely, a diet lacking in these components can lead to an imbalanced microbiota, known as dysbiosis, which has been linked to inflammation and various chronic diseases.

Anti-inflammatory Diets: More Than a Trend

In this context, anti-inflammatory diets are not merely a trend but reflect a scientific understanding of how the foods we eat affect our body. The Mediterranean diet, the DASH diet (Dietary Approaches to Stop Hypertension), and other diets rich in fruits, vegetables, healthy fats, and lean proteins have been shown to reduce inflammation levels.

Preparation for Detailed Analysis

With this understanding of the relationship between diet and inflammation, the next step will be to examine specific food groups and how they influence inflammation. In the following section, we will focus on foods that exacerbate inflammation, identifying which ones to avoid or limit to promote better health and well-being.

2.2 Foods That Exacerbate Inflammation

After understanding the link between diet and inflammation, it's essential to identify specific foods that can exacerbate inflammation. This awareness is crucial for making informed dietary decisions. In the next section, we will focus on foods that mitigate inflammation, but first, let's examine those to limit or avoid.

Refined Sugars and Inflammation

Refined sugars are among the biggest culprits of dietary inflammation. Found abundantly in sweets, sugary beverages, and many processed foods, these sugars can trigger a spike in insulin levels and promote inflammation. Studies have linked high consumption of refined sugars to increased inflammation, obesity, and chronic diseases.

Trans Fats and Inflammation

Trans fats, often present in fried foods, packaged snacks, and commercial baked goods, are known for their inflammatory potential. These fats can alter the lipid balance in the blood, promoting inflammation and increasing the risk of cardiovascular diseases. Avoiding or drastically reducing the intake of these fats is crucial for an anti-inflammatory diet.

High Glycemic Carbohydrates

High glycemic carbohydrates, like white bread, refined pasta, and some breakfast cereals, can cause rapid spikes in blood sugar levels, triggering an inflammatory process. Preferring low glycemic carbohydrates, which provide a slower and more stable release of energy, is a better strategy for controlling inflammation.

Processed Foods and Preservatives

Processed foods often contain preservatives, coloring, and additives that can contribute to inflammation. These compounds can alter gut flora and stimulate inflammatory responses in the body. A diet focused on fresh and minimally processed foods helps reduce the intake of these pro-inflammatory compounds.

Excessive Alcohol

While moderate consumption of certain forms of alcohol, like red wine, may have health benefits, excessive alcohol use is clearly linked to inflammation. Excess alcohol can damage the liver and other organs, stimulating inflammation and compromising overall health.

Next Steps: Anti-inflammatory Foods

Now that we've identified the foods to limit in order to reduce inflammation, the next section will focus on anti-inflammatory foods. This section will provide insights on how to effectively incorporate these foods into your daily diet, countering the effects of pro-inflammatory foods and promoting health and well-being.

2.3 Foods That Reduce Inflammation

After examining foods that can exacerbate inflammation, it's time to focus on those that have the opposite effect. Anti-inflammatory foods play a crucial role in reducing chronic inflammation and promoting overall health. This section deliberates on such foods, providing guidance on how to integrate them into the daily diet, and acting as a bridge to the next section that addresses the principles of an anti-inflammatory diet.

Green Leafy Vegetables

Green leafy vegetables, such as spinach, kale, and Swiss chard, are rich in antioxidants and essential nutrients. They contain vitamins like C and E, and minerals like iron and calcium, which have anti-inflammatory properties. Additionally, their high concentration of phytonutrients, such as chlorophyll, can help reduce inflammation in the body.

Fruits Rich in Antioxidants

Fruits like berries, cherries, and pomegranates are known for their high antioxidant content. These compounds, such as anthocyanins in berries, help neutralize free radicals in the body, reducing inflammation and protecting cells from damage.

Healthy Fats: Omega-3 and Olive Oil

Omega-3 fatty acids, found abundantly in fatty fish like salmon and mackerel, and in seeds like chia and flaxseed, are potent anti-inflammatories. Extra virgin olive oil, another healthy fat, contains oleocanthal, a compound that has been shown to have properties similar to ibuprofen, an anti-inflammatory drug.

Whole Foods and Fiber

Whole foods, such as whole grains, legumes, and vegetables, are rich in fiber. Dietary fibers not only aid digestion but can also modulate the gut microbiota, which in turn can influence inflammation. A healthy gut is crucial for an efficient immune system and for managing inflammation.

Spices and Herbs

Spices like turmeric, ginger, and garlic are not only rich in flavor but also have anti-inflammatory properties. Curcumin, the active ingredient in turmeric, is particularly noted for its powerful anti-inflammatory and antioxidant properties.

Transition to the Next Section

Understanding the importance of these anti-inflammatory foods, the next step is to construct a diet that effectively incorporates them. Section 2.4 will discuss the principles of an anti-inflammatory diet, offering practical advice on how to integrate these foods into daily life and create a balanced and sustainable meal plan.

2.4 Principles of an Anti-Inflammatory Diet

After exploring foods that exacerbate and those that reduce inflammation, it's time to integrate this knowledge into a coherent framework: the principles of an anti-inflammatory diet. This section provides guidelines on how to structure a diet that not only fights inflammation but also promotes overall health and well-being. These principles will serve as the foundation for the next section, which introduces weekly meal plans.

Balance Macronutrients

An anti-inflammatory diet starts with a balance of macronutrients: proteins, fats, and carbohydrates. Proteins should come from lean and high-quality sources, such as fish, poultry, legumes, and tofu. Healthy fats, like those found in olive oil, nuts, and fatty fish, should replace saturated and trans fats. Carbohydrates should primarily come from whole, fiber-rich sources, such as whole grains, fruits, and vegetables.

Increase Antioxidant Intake

Antioxidants are crucial in the fight against inflammation. A diet rich in colorful fruits and vegetables ensures a broad supply of antioxidants. Foods like berries, apples, carrots, spinach, and bell peppers are excellent choices to increase antioxidant intake.

Incorporate Omega-3 Fatty Acids

Omega-3 fatty acids are among the most potent natural anti-inflammatories. Regularly including sources of omega-3, such as fatty fish (salmon, mackerel), flaxseeds, chia seeds, and walnuts, is crucial in an anti-inflammatory diet.

Reduce Processed Food Intake

Processed foods often contain high levels of added sugars, unhealthy fats, and additives that can stimulate inflammation. Limiting or eliminating these foods is a fundamental step towards an anti-inflammatory diet.

Moderate Alcohol Consumption

While moderate alcohol consumption can be part of a balanced diet, it's important to moderate intake. Excess alcohol can contribute to inflammation and other health issues.

Adequate Hydration

Drinking plenty of water is essential for supporting all bodily processes, including reducing inflammation. Adequate hydration helps flush toxins from the body and keeps cells healthy.

Avoid Food Triggers

Identifying and avoiding foods that trigger personal inflammation is important. This can vary from person to person, with some finding dairy products, gluten, or other specific foods can exacerbate inflammation.

Transition to the Next Section

With these principles in mind, we are now ready to move on to constructing anti-inflammatory weekly meal plans. In the next section, we will focus on how to apply these guidelines in practice, developing meal plans that not only reduce inflammation but are also delicious, satisfying, and easy to follow.

2.5 Introduction to Anti-Inflammatory Weekly Meal Plans

Having established the foundational principles of an anti-inflammatory diet, it's time to translate these theories into concrete actions. Anti-inflammatory weekly meal plans represent a practical approach to incorporating foods and habits that reduce inflammation into daily life. This section of the book not only provides examples of meal plans but also offers tips for personalizing them according to individual needs, serving as an ideal link to the next chapter that will focus on specific anti-inflammatory food groups.

Creating Balanced Meal Plans

An effective weekly meal plan should include a wide variety of anti-inflammatory foods, ensuring a balance between proteins, carbohydrates, and healthy fats. Each meal should incorporate vegetables, a source of lean protein, and a fiber-rich element, such as whole grains or legumes. Varying foods is also important to ensure a broad range of nutrients and maintain interest in the meal plan.

Weekly Menu Examples

An example of a weekly menu might include:

- Monday: breakfast with whole oatmeal, berries, and chia seeds; lunch with quinoa salad, spinach, and grilled salmon; dinner with baked chicken breast, steamed broccoli, and sweet potatoes.

- Tuesday: breakfast with a spinach, banana, and almond milk smoothie; lunch with a turkey and vegetable wrap on whole-grain bread; dinner with a lentil and vegetable stew.

And so on for the rest of the week, alternating meals to ensure variety and balance.

Meal Prep Tips

Meal prepping in advance can simplify adhering to a weekly meal plan. Spending a few hours during the weekend to cook and store meals can save time during the week and help avoid less healthy food choices.

Customization According to Individual Needs

Adapting the meal plan to personal needs is important, considering any allergies, intolerances, or preferences. For example, those following a vegetarian or vegan diet can replace animal proteins with plant-based alternatives like tofu, tempeh, or legumes.

Instructions for Gradually Modifying the Diet

For those new to the anti-inflammatory diet, starting with small changes, such as replacing processed snacks with fruit or incorporating more vegetables into meals, can be helpful. This gradual approach eases the transition and makes the change more sustainable in the long term.

Transition to the Next Chapter

Having provided an introduction to anti-inflammatory weekly meal plans, the next chapter will delve into specific anti-inflammatory food groups, such as leafy green vegetables, discussing in detail their health benefits and how to effectively incorporate them into the diet. This natural progression from the general to the specific will help readers understand not only how to build their meal plans but also the reasons behind the selection of specific foods.

Chapter 3: Key Anti-Inflammatory Foods

3.1 Benefits of Leafy Green Vegetables

Initiating the third chapter, we focus on the first group of anti-inflammatory foods: leafy green vegetables. These vegetables are a foundational pillar of an anti-inflammatory diet, thanks to their nutritional density and numerous health benefits. In this section, we delve into the benefits of leafy green vegetables, establishing a basis for discussing other anti-inflammatory foods in subsequent sections.

Nutrient Richness

Leafy green vegetables, such as spinach, kale, Swiss chard, and romaine lettuce, are packed with vitamins, minerals, and fiber, yet low in calories. They are excellent sources of vitamins A, C, E, K, as well as essential minerals like iron, calcium, and potassium. These nutrients support a wide range of bodily functions, from eye health to blood clotting and immune function.

Powerful Antioxidants

These vegetables are loaded with antioxidants, which help combat free radicals in the body, reducing oxidative stress and inflammation. Phytonutrients like lutein and zeaxanthin, abundantly found in leafy greens, are particularly known for their beneficial effects on eye health and in preventing chronic diseases.

Anti-inflammatory Effects

Leafy green vegetables contain natural compounds that have been shown to reduce inflammation in the body. These include flavonoids, carotenoids, and phenolic acids. Regular consumption of these vegetables can help mitigate chronic inflammation and reduce the risk of associated diseases, such as heart disease and diabetes.

Gut Health Support

The fiber in leafy green vegetables supports digestive and gut health. A fiber-rich diet helps regulate bowel movements and can promote a healthy gut microbiome, which plays a crucial role in modulating inflammation and immunity.

Culinary Versatility

Leafy green vegetables are incredibly versatile in the kitchen. They can be eaten raw in salads, blended into smoothies, steamed, sautéed, or added to soups and stews. This versatility makes them an easy and tasty addition to any meal plan.

Transition to the Next Section

After examining the benefits of leafy green vegetables, the next section will focus on another powerful group of foods in the fight against inflammation: berries. We will explore the antioxidant properties of berries and how their inclusion in the diet can offer further anti-inflammatory benefits and promote overall health.

3.2 Antioxidant Power of Berries

Continuing our exploration of anti-inflammatory foods, section 3.2 is dedicated to berries, a group of fruits known for their extraordinary antioxidant properties. This section of the book examines how regular consumption of berries can contribute to reducing inflammation and improving overall health, providing a natural transition to the next section that addresses the importance of healthy fats like olive oil and omega-3-rich fish.

Variety and Nutritional Richness

Berries, such as strawberries, blueberries, raspberries, and blackcurrants, are among the most nutrient-dense fruits available. Rich in vitamins, minerals, and fiber, they have a low-calorie content but are high in nutrients. They are excellent sources of vitamin C, vitamin K, manganese, and dietary fiber.

High Antioxidant Content

Berries are particularly noted for their high antioxidant content, especially anthocyanins, which give them their vibrant color. These antioxidants help neutralize free radicals in the body, reducing inflammation and protecting cells from damage. Research has shown that anthocyanins can have beneficial effects on heart health and may help prevent some chronic diseases.

Effects on Metabolism and Inflammation Reduction

Berries have been shown to positively influence metabolism, helping to improve insulin response and reduce blood sugar levels. This effect is particularly beneficial in managing type 2 diabetes and obesity, conditions often accompanied by chronic inflammation.

Support for Brain Health

Regular consumption of berries has been linked to benefits for brain health. The antioxidants in berries can delay age-related cognitive decline and improve brain function. Moreover, some research suggests that berries may play a role in preventing neurodegenerative diseases like Alzheimer's.

Incorporating Berries into the Diet

Berries can be easily incorporated into the daily diet. They are delicious on their own, in smoothies, salads, yogurt, or as part of healthy desserts. Frozen berries are also a good option, as they retain most of their nutrients and antioxidants.

Transition to the Next Section

Having explored the antioxidant and anti-inflammatory potential of berries, the next section will focus on another crucial group of anti-inflammatory foods: healthy fats. We will examine how olive oil and omega-3-rich fish can not only reduce inflammation but also offer a myriad of other health benefits, thus linking nutritional information with practical recommendations for an optimal anti-inflammatory diet.

3.3 The Importance of Healthy Fats (Olive Oil, Omega-3)

Section 3.3 delves into the essential role of healthy fats, particularly olive oil and omega-3-rich fish, in combating inflammation. This section emphasizes how integrating healthy fats into the diet can not only help reduce inflammation but also promote overall health, linking to the next section that will address spices and herbs with anti-inflammatory properties.

Benefits of Olive Oil

Extra virgin olive oil is a cornerstone of the Mediterranean diet, renowned for its numerous health benefits, especially its anti-inflammatory impact. Rich in monounsaturated fatty acids and phenolic compounds such as oleocanthal, olive oil helps reduce inflammation and protect against heart disease, certain types of cancer, and age-related cognitive decline. Oleocanthal, in particular, has been shown to have effects similar to non-steroidal anti-inflammatory drugs, reducing inflammation in a manner akin to ibuprofen.

Omega-3 in Fatty Fish

Fatty fish like salmon, mackerel, and sardines are excellent sources of omega-3 fatty acids, particularly EPA (eicosapentaenoic acid) and DHA (docosahexaenoic acid). Omega-3s are known for their potent anti-inflammatory properties, which can aid in the prevention and treatment of chronic inflammatory diseases such as rheumatoid arthritis, heart disease, and depression. They reduce inflammation by acting on various biochemical pathways in the body, including decreasing the production of inflammatory chemicals.

Effects on Metabolism and Cardiovascular Health

Healthy fats play a significant role in regulating metabolism, improving endothelial function, and reducing the risk of atherosclerosis. Olive oil and omega-3s help maintain low levels of LDL ("bad") cholesterol and elevate HDL ("good") cholesterol, promoting optimal cardiovascular health.

Incorporating Healthy Fats into the Diet

Olive oil can be used as a dressing for salads, for cooking, or as a substitute for butter. Fatty fish can be integrated into the diet by consuming them at least twice a week, whether grilled, baked, or steamed. For those who do not consume fish, fish oil or algae supplements can be a useful alternative to obtain the necessary omega-3s.

Attention to Sources and Quality

It's important to choose high-quality extra virgin olive oil to maximize health benefits. Similarly, for fatty fish, opting for sustainable sources and those low in mercury is preferable.

Transition to the Next Section

After examining the critical role of healthy fats, the next section will focus on spices and herbs. These not only add flavor to our dishes but can also offer significant anti-inflammatory benefits. We will explore how ingredients like turmeric, ginger, and garlic can be incorporated into the daily diet to maximize their health effects.

3.4 Spices and Herbs with Anti-inflammatory Properties

Continuing our exploration of anti-inflammatory foods, section 3.4 focuses on spices and herbs. These ingredients not only enrich the flavor of our dishes but also offer significant anti-inflammatory benefits. This section explores how incorporating specific spices and herbs into the diet can help combat inflammation, serving as a bridge to the next section that will discuss integrating these foods into the daily diet.

Turmeric: A Powerful Anti-inflammatory

Turmeric, with its active component, curcumin, is one of the most renowned spices for its anti-inflammatory properties. Extensive research has shown that curcumin can reduce inflammation in various chronic conditions, such as arthritis, heart disease, and intestinal disorders. It is also a potent antioxidant, contributing to reducing oxidative stress in the body.

Ginger: Beyond Nausea Relief

Ginger is another spice with strong anti-inflammatory properties. Traditionally used to alleviate nausea, ginger has also been shown to reduce muscle pain, joint inflammation, and symptoms of some autoimmune diseases. Its bioactive compounds, like gingerol, have anti-inflammatory and antioxidant effects.

Garlic: Natural Power Against Inflammation

Garlic, known for its antimicrobial properties, is also a potent anti-inflammatory. It contains compounds like allicin, which have been shown to reduce markers of inflammation in the body. Garlic also supports cardiovascular health, helping to lower blood pressure and cholesterol.

Other Anti-inflammatory Herbs and Spices

There are many other herbs and spices that can help reduce inflammation, including cinnamon, rosemary, thyme, and oregano. Each of these contains unique combinations of antioxidant and anti-inflammatory compounds that can contribute to optimal health.

Incorporating into Daily Recipes

Spices and herbs can be easily incorporated into daily cooking. Turmeric can be added to soups, stews, or smoothies. Ginger is great in tea, smoothies, or marinades. Garlic can be used in virtually any savory dish, while herbs like rosemary and thyme are excellent for flavoring meats, vegetables, and sauces.

Attention to Interactions and Contraindications

Although these spices and herbs are generally safe, it's important to consider any interactions with medications or existing medical conditions. For example, high doses of turmeric can interfere with some blood-thinning medications.

Transition to the Next Section

After exploring the importance of anti-inflammatory spices and herbs, the next section will focus on how to integrate all these anti-inflammatory foods - leafy green vegetables, berries, healthy fats, spices, and herbs - into the daily diet. We'll provide practical tips and meal ideas that incorporate these powerful ingredients, helping readers create a comprehensive and effective dietary regimen against inflammation.

3.5 Integrating Anti-inflammatory Foods into the Daily Diet

After reviewing a variety of anti-inflammatory foods, from the power of leafy greens to the beneficial properties of spices, section 3.5 focuses on how to effectively incorporate these foods into the daily diet. This integration is crucial for maximizing their anti-inflammatory benefits, creating a comprehensive and varied dietary approach. These integration strategies will serve as the foundation for the next chapter, which addresses avoiding pro-inflammatory foods.

Creating a Dietary Balance

A balanced approach to the anti-inflammatory diet includes a mix of leafy green vegetables, fruits like berries, sources of healthy fats, and a wide variety of spices and herbs. The goal is to create dishes that are not only nutritious but also delicious and satisfying, to ensure that this diet is sustainable in the long term.

Breakfast Ideas

Start your day with a breakfast that incorporates anti-inflammatory foods:

- Green smoothies with spinach, blueberries, and flaxseed.

- Oatmeal porridge with a sprinkle of cinnamon, blueberries, and nuts.

- Frittata with green vegetables and a touch of garlic and turmeric.

Lunch and Dinner Tips

For lunches and dinners, focus on dishes that include a variety of anti-inflammatory components:

- Rich salads with a base of leafy greens, addition of salmon or tuna for omega-3s, and a dressing made of olive oil and lemon.

- Soups and stews that include ginger, turmeric, and garlic, with an abundant assortment of vegetables and legumes.

- Main dishes that include fatty fish or chicken, accompanied by a generous portion of green vegetables and seasoned with fresh herbs.

Healthy Snacks and Desserts

For snacks, choose options that promote health and fight inflammation:

- Fresh fruit like berries or apples, paired with a handful of nuts.

- Raw vegetables with hummus or guacamole based on olive oil.

- Healthy desserts, such as chia pudding with almond milk and berries.

Customization According to Individual Needs

Remember that each individual is unique; therefore, it's important to customize the diet according to personal needs, preferences, and health conditions. Listen to your body and, if necessary, consult a nutritionist for personalized advice.

Transition to the Next Chapter

Having now provided practical advice on incorporating a variety of anti-inflammatory foods into the daily diet, the next chapter will move on to identify and discuss pro-inflammatory foods. This shift in focus from what we should include to what we should limit or avoid is essential for adopting a comprehensive approach to managing inflammation through diet.

Chapter 4: Avoiding Pro-Inflammatory Foods

4.1 Identifying Refined Sugars and Their Effects

In the fourth chapter, we shift from exploring anti-inflammatory foods to the importance of identifying and reducing foods that can worsen inflammation. Section 4.1 focuses on refined sugars, often a hidden and harmful component in the modern diet. This section explores how refined sugars influence inflammation and overall health, laying the groundwork for the next section on the impact of trans fats.

The Pervasiveness of Refined Sugars

Refined sugars are ubiquitous in the modern diet, found in a wide range of products beyond the obvious sweets, such as sugary drinks, breakfast cereals, packaged snacks, and even in some savory products. These sugars, stripped of their fibers and nutrients during the refining process, are rapidly absorbed into the bloodstream, causing spikes in glucose and insulin.

Metabolic Effects

These rapid spikes and drops in blood sugar levels can lead to a range of metabolic problems, including insulin resistance, a precursor to type 2 diabetes. Moreover, high consumption of refined sugars is often linked to weight gain and obesity, both associated with increased inflammation in the body.

Contribution to Chronic Inflammation

Refined sugars stimulate inflammation through several mechanisms. They can induce an increase in blood fatty acid levels and promote the production of pro-inflammatory cytokines, proteins that contribute to systemic inflammation. This chronic inflammatory process has been linked to a variety of diseases, including heart disease, some types of cancer, and autoimmune disorders.

Identifying and Reducing Refined Sugars

To reduce the intake of refined sugars:

- Carefully read food labels to identify hidden sugars.

- Limit the consumption of foods and beverages with added sugars.

- Choose foods in their whole and unprocessed form, such as fresh fruit instead of fruit juices or canned fruit.

- Use natural sweeteners in moderation, like honey or maple syrup, which contain some nutrients and are less refined.

Transition to the Next Section

After understanding the role of refined sugars in exacerbating inflammation and the steps to reduce their consumption, the next section will examine another problematic group of foods: trans fats. We will explore how trans fats negatively impact health and why it is essential to minimize or eliminate their consumption for an effective anti-inflammatory diet.

4.2 The Impact of Trans Fats on Health

Continuing the discussion on foods that exacerbate inflammation, section 4.2 focuses on trans fats, known for their negative health effects. This section examines how trans fats influence inflammation and overall health, preparing the reader to better understand the impact of high glycemic index carbohydrates, the subject of the next section.

What Are Trans Fats?

Trans fats are a type of unsaturated fat, often formed through an industrial process of hydrogenation, which turns liquid oils into solids at room temperature. This process is used to improve the shelf life and texture of many packaged foods, such as snacks, commercial baked goods, and fast food.

Negative Effects on Cardiovascular Health

Trans fats are particularly harmful to cardiovascular health. They increase levels of LDL cholesterol ("bad") and reduce HDL cholesterol ("good"), contributing to the formation of plaque in the arteries (atherosclerosis). This can significantly increase the risk of heart disease and stroke.

Contribution to Chronic Inflammation

Beyond their effects on cholesterol, trans fats can promote inflammation. They have been linked to elevated levels of inflammatory markers such as C-reactive protein (CRP), suggesting a direct impact on systemic inflammation. This chronic inflammation is a risk factor for many chronic diseases, including type 2 diabetes.

Reducing Trans Fats in the Diet

To reduce trans fats:

- Avoid or limit the consumption of fried foods and packaged snacks.

- Read nutrition labels carefully and look for terms like "partially hydrogenated oils," an indicator of the presence of trans fats.

- Prefer healthy fats found in olive oil, nuts, and fatty fish.

- Choose homemade or bakery-made baked goods that use healthy oils.

Regulations and Consumer Awareness

Many countries have introduced regulations to limit the use of trans fats in food products. However, consumer awareness is crucial, as some products may still contain them in small amounts.

Transition to the Next Section

After examining the negative impact of trans fats on inflammation and overall health, the next section will address another problematic group of foods: high glycemic index carbohydrates. These carbohydrates can cause spikes in blood sugar, exacerbating inflammation and contributing to various health issues, a topic that is essential to fully understand the importance of a balanced and anti-inflammatory diet.

4.3 Problems with High Glycemic Index Carbohydrates

In section 4.3, we focus on high glycemic index carbohydrates and their role in exacerbating inflammation. This section of the book aims to illustrate how high consumption of these carbohydrates can negatively affect health and promote chronic inflammation, preparing the reader to understand the importance of healthier food choices in the next section.

What Are High Glycemic Index Carbohydrates?

High glycemic index carbohydrates are those that are digested and absorbed quickly, leading to a rapid increase in blood glucose levels. Examples include white bread, potatoes, many breakfast cereals and processed snacks, sweets, and sugary drinks.

Impact on Blood Sugar and Inflammation

When consuming high glycemic index foods, the body must produce large amounts of insulin to manage the sudden spike in blood glucose. These spikes can lead to insulin resistance over time, a condition closely associated with type 2 diabetes and obesity. Moreover, high levels of glucose and insulin are factors that can stimulate chronic inflammation.

Link with Chronic Diseases

Frequent consumption of high glycemic index carbohydrates has been linked to an increased risk of chronic diseases, not just type 2 diabetes but also heart disease and some forms of cancer. These diseases are often characterized by chronic inflammatory states, suggesting a direct link between diet and inflammation.

Strategies to Reduce High Glycemic Index Carbohydrates

To minimize the negative effects of high glycemic index carbohydrates:

- Choose low glycemic index carbohydrates, such as whole grains, legumes, fruits, and vegetables.

- Balance carbohydrates with proteins and healthy fats to slow absorption and reduce blood glucose spikes.

- Avoid processed snacks and pre-packaged foods that often contain large amounts of high glycemic index carbohydrates.

- Be mindful of portions and how carbohydrates are prepared, as these factors can affect the glycemic index.

Transition to the Next Section

Understanding the issues associated with high glycemic index carbohydrates and how they can contribute to inflammation and chronic diseases, the next section will focus on practical advice to reduce the consumption of these foods. We will discuss strategies for making more informed and balanced food choices, including healthy and tasty substitutions, to help prevent or manage inflammation through diet.

4.4 Tips for Reducing Consumption of Pro-Inflammatory Foods

In section 4.4, we focus on practical strategies for reducing the consumption of pro-inflammatory foods, especially those high in glycemic index and rich in trans fats and refined sugars. This section of the book provides practical and accessible advice for making healthier food choices, laying the groundwork for the next section that deals with healthy and tasty substitutions.

Recognizing and Avoiding Pro-Inflammatory Foods

The first step to reducing the consumption of pro-inflammatory foods is recognizing them. These often include processed foods, packaged snacks, sweets, sugary beverages, fried foods, and fast food. Carefully reading nutritional labels and familiarizing yourself with the names of pro-inflammatory ingredients can help make more informed choices.

Healthy Substitutions

Replacing pro-inflammatory foods with healthier alternatives can have a significant impact. Some examples include:

- Swapping refined grains for whole grains, such as choosing whole wheat bread over white bread.

- Opting for natural snacks like fresh fruit, unsalted nuts, or vegetables with hummus instead of packaged snacks.

- Preparing meals at home using fresh and minimally processed ingredients.

The Importance of Home Cooking

Preparing meals at home allows complete control over the ingredients used. Cooking with healthy methods like grilling, steaming, or baking can reduce the use of unhealthy fats and better preserve the nutrients in foods.

Reducing Sweeteners and Added Sugars

A simple way to cut down on refined sugars is to decrease the use of sweeteners in foods and beverages. Consider natural alternatives like stevia or honey, but these should also be used in moderation.

Increasing Whole Food Consumption

Focus on foods in their most whole and natural form. This includes a wide consumption of fruits and vegetables, whole grains, legumes, nuts and seeds, and lean protein sources.

Monitoring Portions

Paying attention to portion sizes can help avoid overconsumption of pro-inflammatory foods. Eating moderate portions, focusing on the quality of foods rather than quantity, can be an effective approach.

Transition to the Next Section

After exploring these strategies for reducing the consumption of pro-inflammatory foods, the next section will examine how to make smart and tasty substitutions in the diet. These substitutions will not only help reduce inflammation but also make the eating experience more enjoyable and sustainable.

4.5 Healthy and Tasty Substitutions

In section 4.5, we focus on how to make healthy and tasty substitutions in the diet, a crucial aspect of reducing the consumption of pro-inflammatory foods without sacrificing the pleasure of eating. This section offers practical ideas for replacing pro-inflammatory foods with healthier alternatives, linking to the next chapter, which will discuss creating a balanced meal plan.

Replacing Refined Carbohydrates

- **Bread and Pasta:** Replace white bread and refined pasta with their whole-grain counterparts, which are richer in fiber and nutrients.

- **White Rice:** Choose brown rice, quinoa, or bulgur, which have a lower glycemic index and are richer in nutrients.

Alternatives to Traditional Sweets

- **Sweeteners:** Use natural sweeteners like honey or maple syrup instead of refined sugar, and reduce the total amount used.

- **Sweet Snacks:** Opt for fresh or dried fruit, Greek yogurt with a touch of honey, or homemade energy bars with natural ingredients.

Substitutions for Unhealthy Fats

- **Cooking with Healthy Oils:** Use extra virgin olive oil or coconut oil instead of butter or margarine for cooking.

- **Frying:** Limit the consumption of fried foods and, when possible, choose cooking methods such as baking, grilling, or steaming.

Healthy Beverages

- **Sugary Drinks:** Replace sugary beverages with naturally flavored water, unsweetened tea, or homemade fruit smoothies.

- **Alcoholic Drinks:** Reduce alcohol consumption and, when you do drink, choose low-calorie options like red wine or light beer.

Reducing Processed Snacks

- **Salty Snacks:** Instead of chips and packaged snacks, choose unsalted nuts, seeds, fresh vegetable sticks, or homemade popcorn without butter.

- **Energy Bars and Cereals:** Opt for options with few added sugars and natural ingredients, or make them at home.

Creative Ideas for Healthy Meals

- **Creative Substitutions:** Use chopped cauliflower as a base for pizza or 'fake' risotto, spiralize zucchini to make vegetable spaghetti, or use lettuce instead of bread for wraps.

- **Experiment in the Kitchen:** Experiment with spices and herbs to add flavor without resorting to excess salt or fats.

Transition to the Next Chapter

With these substitutions, you can enjoy delicious meals while reducing your intake of pro-inflammatory foods. In the next chapter, we'll explore how to create a balanced meal plan, integrating these healthy choices into daily life to form sustainable eating habits that support the fight against inflammation.

Chapter 5: Weekly Meal Plans

5.1 Creating a Balanced Meal Plan

In the fifth chapter, we focus on creating balanced meal plans that incorporate the teachings from the previous chapters. Section 5.1 outlines how to structure a dietary regimen that is anti-inflammatory, nutritious, and sustainable, serving as a foundation for the next section that will present examples of anti-inflammatory weekly menus.

Fundamental Principles of a Balanced Meal Plan

A balanced meal plan should meet the body's nutritional needs, including a variety of foods to ensure a broad intake of essential nutrients.

- **Variety:** Incorporate a wide range of foods to ensure that the body receives all the necessary macro and micronutrients. This includes lean proteins, complex carbohydrates, healthy fats, and an abundance of fruits and vegetables.

- **Macronutrient Balance:** Balance the intake of proteins, carbohydrates, and fats. For example, each meal should contain a source of protein, a serving of complex carbohydrates (such as whole grains or legumes), and a moderate amount of healthy fats.

- **Nutrient Density:** Choose foods that are nutrient-dense rather than calorie-dense. Foods like leafy green vegetables, fresh fruit, nuts, seeds, and fatty fish are excellent choices.

Meal Planning

- **Breakfast:** Start the day with a nutritious breakfast that might include whole-grain oats, Greek yogurt with berries and chia seeds, or eggs with leafy green vegetables.

- **Lunch:** Prepare balanced lunches like rich salads with lean proteins and healthy fats, or soups and stews that include a variety of vegetables.

- **Dinner:** Create dinners that include a serving of lean protein, a generous portion of vegetables, and a source of complex carbohydrates.

Healthy Snacking

- Opt for snacks that sustain energy and nutrition, such as fresh fruit, nuts, vegetables with hummus, or Greek yogurt.

The Importance of Hydration

- Maintaining adequate hydration is crucial. Drinking water, unsweetened tea, and other sugar-free beverages helps support digestion and nutrient absorption.

Listening to Your Body

- It's important to be attentive to your body's signals. Adjusting portions and meal compositions based on hunger, energy, and overall well-being is key to a sustainable meal plan.

Transition to the Next Section

After outlining the principles for creating a balanced meal plan, the next section will present examples of anti-inflammatory weekly menus. These examples will help visualize how different foods can be combined into daily meals to support an effective and enjoyable anti-inflammatory diet.

5.2 Examples of Anti-Inflammatory Weekly Menus

After establishing the principles of a balanced diet, section 5.2 of the book presents concrete examples of anti-inflammatory weekly menus. These menus are designed to illustrate how to integrate various anti-inflammatory foods into delicious and satisfying daily meals, serving as a practical model for readers. These examples facilitate the transition to the next section, which will focus on meal preparation and planning.

Weekly Menu Example

Monday

- **Breakfast:** Spinach, banana, and flaxseed smoothie with almond milk.

- **Lunch:** Quinoa salad with mixed vegetables, avocado, and grilled chicken breast.

- **Dinner:** Baked salmon with asparagus and baked sweet potatoes.

Tuesday

- **Breakfast:** Greek yogurt with fresh blueberries and a sprinkle of nuts.

- **Lunch:** Whole wheat wrap with turkey, lettuce, tomatoes, and hummus.

- **Dinner:** Lentil stew with mixed vegetables and a slice of whole grain bread.

Wednesday

- **Breakfast:** Cooked oatmeal with sliced apples, cinnamon, and a drizzle of honey.

- **Lunch:** Farro salad with cherry tomatoes, cucumbers, olives, and feta.

- **Dinner:** Grilled chicken breast with steamed broccoli and brown rice.

Thursday

- **Breakfast:** Scrambled eggs with spinach and mushrooms, served on whole grain toast.

- **Lunch:** Vegetable soup with a side of mixed salad.

- **Dinner:** Chickpea curry with whole grain basmati rice.

Friday

- **Breakfast:** Oat pancakes with berries and natural maple syrup.

- **Lunch:** Tuna salad with lettuce, tomato, and avocado.

- **Dinner:** Grilled trout fillet with quinoa and sautéed spinach.

Saturday

- **Breakfast:** Smoothie bowl with fresh fruit and chia seeds.

- **Lunch:** Avocado toast on whole grain bread with poached eggs.

- **Dinner:** Lean beef steak with baked sweet potatoes and a green salad.

Sunday

- **Breakfast:** Chia pudding made with almond milk and berries.

- **Lunch:** Greek salad with grilled chicken.

- **Dinner:** Whole wheat spaghetti with homemade marinara sauce and turkey meatballs.

Tips for Variety

It's important to vary meals to avoid monotony and ensure a broad intake of different nutrients. Experimenting with different vegetables, protein sources, and whole grains can make meals more interesting and nutritious.

Transition to the Next Section

Having provided examples of how to incorporate anti-inflammatory foods into a weekly meal plan, the next section will focus on meal preparation. We'll discuss how to organize the kitchen and prepare meals in advance to simplify adherence to an anti-inflammatory diet and make the process more manageable and less time-consuming.

5.3 Meal Prep Tips

This chapter delves into essential strategies for sustaining an anti-inflammatory diet through organized meal preparation. This section provides practical advice for planning and preparing meals ahead of time, ensuring adherence to a healthy and balanced eating plan. These tips set the stage for the next discussion on adapting the diet to specific dietary needs.

Planning and Organization:

- **Weekly Meal Planning:** Allocating time each week to plan meals helps avoid impulsive food choices and ensures that meals are balanced and in line with dietary objectives.

- **Shopping List:** Creating a shopping list based on meal plans ensures all necessary ingredients are purchased, reducing the need for last-minute supermarket trips.

Advance Preparation:

- **Batch Cooking:** Preparing large quantities of staples, such as whole grains, legumes, or proteins, for use in various meals throughout the week.

- **Ready-to-Use Vegetables:** Washing, cutting, and storing vegetables immediately after purchase simplifies meal preparation.

- **Sauces and Dressings:** Preparing healthy sauces and dressings ahead of time to quickly enhance meals.

Storage and Freezing:

- **Quality Containers:** Investing in high-quality food containers, preferably glass, for meal storage in the fridge or freezer.

- **Portioning:** Storing meals in individual portions facilitates portion control and the selection of a quick and healthy meal option.

Versatile and Creative Cooking:

- **Flexible Recipes:** Choosing recipes that can be easily adjusted based on available ingredients. This minimizes waste and adds variety to the diet.

- **Creative Cooking:** Experimenting with different spices, herbs, and marinades to diversify flavors without adding pro-inflammatory ingredients.

Time and Energy Management:

- **Cook When Convenient:** Utilizing times during the week when you have more time or energy for cooking, such as the weekend, to prepare meals in advance.

- **Multi-tasking Cooking:** Using pressure cookers, slow cookers, or ovens to prepare multiple dishes simultaneously, saving time and energy.

Transitioning to the Next Topic:

After examining effective meal organization and preparation strategies, the next section of the book will explore adapting the anti-inflammatory diet to specific dietary needs, such as allergies, intolerances, or personal preferences. This personalized approach ensures the anti-inflammatory diet is not only effective but also enjoyable and suited to individual circumstances.

5.4 Adaptations for Specific Dietary Needs

Section 5.4 of the book discusses the importance of customizing the anti-inflammatory diet based on each individual's specific dietary needs, whether they're dictated by health conditions, allergies, food intolerances, or personal preferences. This customization is crucial to ensure that the diet is not only healthy but also sustainable and enjoyable, a concept that will be further developed in section 5.5, which discusses maintaining variety and flavor.

Considerations for Allergies and Intolerances

- **Substitutions for Allergies:** For those with allergies to certain foods, it's important to find suitable substitutions that do not compromise nutritional or anti-inflammatory value. For example, if allergic to seafood, seek alternative sources of omega-3s in flaxseeds or chia seeds.

- **Managing Food Intolerances:** For intolerances such as lactose or gluten, choosing alternatives like lactose-free dairy products or gluten-free grains can be crucial.

Adaptations for a Vegetarian or Vegan Diet

- **Plant-based Proteins:** For vegetarians and vegans, incorporating a variety of plant-based protein sources such as legumes, tofu, tempeh, and seitan is important.

- **Nutritional Supplementation:** Ensure the intake of essential nutrients that may be less available in a plant-based diet, such as B12, iron, calcium, omega-3s, and vitamin D.

Considerations for Specific Health Conditions

- **Diabetes:** For those with diabetes, focusing on low glycemic index foods and monitoring carbohydrate intake to manage blood sugar levels is key.

- **Heart Disease:** For those with heart conditions, limiting saturated and trans fats while increasing the intake of healthy fats like those found in olive oil and fatty fish is advisable.

Strategies for Weight Loss

- **Portion Control:** If weight loss is the goal, portion control can be a crucial aspect. Using smaller plates and listening to the body's satiety signals can help.

- **Low-Calorie Choices:** Prefer nutrient-rich, low-calorie foods like vegetables and fruits to increase meal volume without excessive calories.

Transition to the Next Section

After examining how to adapt an anti-inflammatory diet to specific needs, the next section will address how to maintain variety and taste in the dietary regimen. This is essential to ensure that the anti-inflammatory diet not only supports health but also remains a pleasurable and rewarding culinary experience.

5.5 Maintaining Variety and Flavor

Section 5.5 of the book is dedicated to how to maintain variety and flavor in an anti-inflammatory diet, a fundamental aspect to ensure that this dietary regime is not only healthy but also enjoyable and gratifying. This section lays the groundwork for the next chapter, which will explore the importance of integrating other lifestyle aspects, such as exercise and stress management, in supporting the immune system and reducing inflammation.

Exploring a Variety of Foods

- **Experimentation:** Try new foods and recipes regularly. Explore different ethnic cuisines that offer a wide variety of anti-inflammatory dishes, such as Mediterranean or Asian cuisine.

- **Seasonality:** Choose seasonal foods to ensure they are at their peak of freshness and flavor. Seasonal foods are often more nutritious and tastier.

Creative Cooking Techniques

- **Cooking Methods:** Experiment with different cooking techniques such as roasting, grilling, steaming, or stir-frying to enhance the natural flavors of foods.

- **Marinades and Dressings:** Use marinades, spices, herbs, and healthy dressings to add flavor without adding calories or pro-inflammatory substances.

Using Spices and Herbs

- **Aromatic Herbs:** Incorporate fresh or dried herbs abundantly, like basil, cilantro, rosemary, and thyme, to enrich dishes.

- **Spices:** Spices not only add flavor but can also offer anti-inflammatory benefits. Use turmeric, ginger, garlic, cinnamon, and other spices to add depth and complexity to your dishes.

Balanced Recipes and Meals

- **Recipe Creativity:** Experiment with recipes that combine different food groups, such as rich salads, nutritious soups, and balanced one-dish meals.

- **Tasty Substitutes:** For desserts, choose healthier options like fresh fruit with Greek yogurt or chia pudding, satisfying the sweet tooth without added sugars.

Engaging All the Senses

- **Plate Presentation:** Presentation can influence how we perceive food. Serve dishes attractively to make the meal experience more enjoyable.

- **Eating Experience:** Eating should be an experience that involves all the senses, not just taste. Enjoy the appearance, smell, and texture of foods, in addition to their flavor.

Transition to the Next Chapter

Maintaining variety and flavor is essential for a sustainable and enjoyable anti-inflammatory diet. In the next chapter, we'll explore how other lifestyle aspects, including regular exercise and stress management, are equally important in supporting the immune system and reducing chronic inflammation.

Chapter 6: Beyond Diet - An Anti-inflammatory Lifestyle

6.1 The Importance of Physical Activity

Section 6.1 explores how physical activity is an essential component in managing and reducing chronic inflammation, enriching the framework of an anti-inflammatory lifestyle that goes beyond diet. This section lays the groundwork for the next section, which will discuss the role of adequate sleep in supporting the immune system and reducing inflammation.

Role of Physical Exercise in Inflammation

- **Reduction of Inflammatory Markers:** Regular physical activity can significantly reduce inflammatory markers in the body, such as C-reactive protein (CRP) and interleukin-6.

- **Metabolic Improvement:** Physical activity helps improve metabolism and insulin sensitivity, reducing the risk of conditions that can be associated with chronic inflammation, like type 2 diabetes and obesity.

Recommended Types of Exercise

- **Aerobic Exercise:** Activities like walking, running, swimming, or cycling help improve cardiovascular health and reduce inflammation.

- **Strength Training:** Strength training, such as weight lifting or using resistance bands, helps build and maintain muscle mass, which is important for regulating inflammation.

- **Flexibility and Balance Exercises:** Activities like yoga or pilates can reduce stress, another key factor in chronic inflammation.

Frequency and Intensity

- **General Recommendations:** Adults should aim for about 150 minutes of moderate-intensity aerobic activity per week, along with two days of muscle-strengthening activities.

- **Customization:** The intensity and type of exercise should be adapted to individual capabilities, health conditions, and fitness levels.

Psychological Benefits of Exercise

- **Stress Reduction:** Physical exercise is a powerful stress reducer, helping to decrease the production of stress hormones, which can exacerbate inflammation.

- **Improved Mood and Sleep:** Regular physical activity can improve sleep quality and mood, providing additional benefits in managing inflammation.

Strategies to Maintain Regularity

- **Incorporate Activity into Daily Routine:** Find ways to include exercise in everyday life, such as walking during lunch breaks or using the stairs instead of the elevator.

- **Enjoyable Activities:** Choosing forms of exercise that you enjoy increases the likelihood of adhering to a regular routine.

Transition to the Next Section

Having established the importance of physical exercise in reducing inflammation and improving overall health, the next section will examine another essential pillar of an anti-inflammatory lifestyle: adequate sleep. We will explore how quality sleep can influence the immune system and contribute to the management of inflammation.

6.2 The Role of Sleep in Managing Inflammation

Section 6.2 addresses the importance of adequate sleep in managing inflammation, highlighting how good sleep hygiene is crucial for the optimal functioning of the immune system. This section connects the topic of sleep with the next, which will discuss stress management techniques, another vital aspect in controlling inflammation.

Impact of Sleep on Inflammation

- **Immune Regulation:** During sleep, the body performs essential repair and regeneration functions. Insufficient or poor-quality sleep can impair the immune system's ability to regulate inflammation.

- **Inflammatory Markers:** Lack of sleep has been linked to increases in inflammatory markers, such as C-reactive protein (CRP) and interleukin-6.

Quantity and Quality of Sleep

- **Recommended Duration:** Adults should aim for 7-9 hours of sleep per night. Regularly getting less than 6 hours of sleep is often associated with increased inflammation.

- **Sleep Quality:** It's not just the quantity, but also the quality of sleep that matters. Deep, uninterrupted sleep is crucial for physical and mental well-being.

Improving Sleep Hygiene

- **Evening Routine:** Establishing a relaxing evening routine can help prepare the body and mind for sleep, such as reading a book or taking a warm bath.

- **Sleep Environment:** Keep the bedroom quiet, dark, and cool, and use comfortable mattresses and pillows.

- **Limiting Blue Light Exposure:** Reduce exposure to blue light from electronic device screens before bedtime, as it can disrupt circadian rhythms and make it harder to fall asleep.

Connection Between Diet, Exercise, and Sleep

- **Diet and Sleep:** Avoid heavy meals, caffeine, and alcohol close to bedtime, as they can disturb sleep.

- **Exercise and Sleep:** Regular exercise can improve sleep quality and duration, but it's best to avoid intense physical activities in the evening hours.

Managing Sleep Disorders

- **Identifying and Treating Sleep Disorders:** Conditions such as insomnia or sleep apnea should be appropriately addressed, consulting a healthcare provider if necessary.

Transition to the Next Section

After examining the importance of sleep in managing inflammation, the next section will explore how effective stress management is another fundamental aspect. Stress reduction techniques not only improve sleep quality but also have a direct impact on reducing chronic inflammation.

6.3 Stress Management Techniques

Section 6.3 focuses on stress management techniques, a vital aspect in reducing chronic inflammation and improving overall health. This section outlines how stress influences inflammation and provides practical strategies for managing it, setting the stage for the next section that will examine how to avoid harmful environmental and lifestyle factors.

Impact of Stress on Inflammation

- **Stress-Inflammation Correlation:** Chronic stress can increase the production of stress hormones such as cortisol and adrenaline, which can in turn stimulate inflammatory processes in the body.

- **Stress and the Immune System:** Elevated and prolonged levels of stress can weaken the immune system, making the body more susceptible to inflammation and illness.

Stress Reduction Techniques

- **Mindfulness and Meditation:** Practices of mindfulness and meditation can reduce stress and improve emotional response to external stimuli.

- **Breathing Exercises:** Deep breathing techniques help calm the nervous system and can be utilized in moments of acute stress.

- **Yoga:** Yoga combines physical movement, controlled breathing, and meditation, making it an effective tool in stress management.

Establishing Relaxing Routines

- **Daily Routine:** Incorporate relaxing activities into the daily routine, such as reading, taking a warm bath, or listening to calm music.

- **Time in Nature:** Spending time outdoors and in nature can significantly reduce stress and improve mood.

Time Management and Delegation

- **Organization and Planning:** Use time management techniques to avoid overload and stress due to commitments and deadlines.

- **Delegating Responsibilities:** Learn to delegate tasks when possible to reduce workload and stress.

Social Support

- **Community and Relationships:** Maintaining positive social relationships and seeking support from friends and family can offer significant relief from stress.

- **Professional Counseling:** For chronic stress or anxiety, consider seeking help from a professional.

Transition to the Next Section

Having discussed the importance of stress management and techniques to achieve it, the next section will examine how to avoid environmental and lifestyle factors that can contribute to inflammation. This includes choosing safer products for home and work, as well as adopting lifestyle habits that support overall health.

6.4 Avoiding Harmful Environmental and Lifestyle Factors

In section 6.4, we delve into the importance of avoiding or minimizing exposure to environmental and lifestyle factors that can contribute to chronic inflammation. This section offers advice on making informed choices that can reduce exposure to these harmful factors, setting the stage for the next section, which will discuss creating an anti-inflammatory daily routine.

Identifying Harmful Environmental Factors

- **Pollutants and Chemicals:** Be mindful of potentially harmful chemicals present in the environment, such as air pollutants, pesticides, and chemical additives in food and household products.

- **Reducing Exposure:** Use water filters, choose organic foods when possible, and prefer household and personal care products with natural ingredients and without harsh chemicals.

Lifestyle Impact

- **Smoking and Alcohol Consumption:** Avoid smoking and limit alcohol consumption, both known for their pro-inflammatory effects.

- **Weight Management:** Maintaining a healthy body weight is important, as obesity can be a contributing factor to inflammation.

Healthy Lifestyle Choices

- **Regular Physical Activity:** As discussed in previous sections, physical activity is essential in reducing inflammation.

- **Balanced Diet:** Continue following an anti-inflammatory diet rich in whole foods, vegetables, fruits, and healthy fats.

Home and Work Environment

- **Healthy Living and Working Spaces:** Create home and work environments that support a healthy lifestyle, such as well-ventilated spaces, with plants, natural light, and quiet zones for relaxation.

- **Reducing Exposure to Electromagnetic Radiation:** Limit time spent in front of screens and electronic devices, especially before bedtime.

Relaxation and Leisure Time

- **Hobbies and Interests:** Engage in relaxing activities and hobbies that reduce stress and promote overall well-being.

- **Time in Nature:** Spending time outdoors, in natural environments, can have a positive effect on reducing stress and inflammation.

Transition to the Next Section

After exploring how to avoid harmful environmental and lifestyle factors, the next section will focus on creating an anti-inflammatory daily routine. This routine will include practical tips on integrating healthy habits into everyday life, emphasizing the importance of a holistic approach in managing inflammation.

6.5 Creating an Anti-Inflammatory Daily Routine

Section 6.5 of the book focuses on creating an anti-inflammatory daily routine, a holistic approach integrating dietary, physical, and mental practices discussed in previous chapters. This section offers practical advice for incorporating daily habits that can help reduce inflammation, serving as an introduction to the next chapter that will explore the importance of a holistic approach to life for lasting well-being.

Starting the Day Healthily

- **Nutritious Breakfast:** Begin the day with an anti-inflammatory breakfast, such as a berry and chia seed smoothie or oatmeal with fruit and nuts.

- **Light Morning Exercise:** Engage in light physical activity, like yoga, stretching, or a brief walk, to stimulate circulation and overall well-being.

Incorporating Movement Throughout the Day

- **Active Breaks:** Integrate short movement breaks throughout the day, especially if leading a sedentary lifestyle.

- **Breathing Exercises:** Use breathing techniques to manage moments of stress and maintain calmness.

Mindful Eating

- **Smart Food Choices:** Maintain a mindful approach to food choices, favoring anti-inflammatory foods and avoiding pro-inflammatory ones.

- **Hydration:** Drink plenty of water throughout the day to aid digestion and toxin elimination.

Stress Management and Evening Relaxation

- **Relaxation Techniques:** Practice evening relaxation techniques, such as reading, taking a warm bath, or meditating, to prepare the body and mind for sleep.
- **Limiting Technology Exposure:** Reduce the use of electronic devices before bedtime to improve sleep quality.

Integrating Healthy Practices

- **Mindfulness:** Practice mindfulness throughout the day to increase awareness and reduce stress reactivity.

- **Creative Activities and Hobbies:** Allocate time for hobbies and creative activities that help divert the mind from daily worries and promote mental well-being.

Regular Health Check-ups

- **Health Monitoring:** Keep track of your health with regular check-ups, especially if you have pre-existing conditions related to inflammation.

- **Listening to Your Body:** Be attentive to your body's signals and make adjustments to your routine as needed.

Transition to the Next Chapter

With these components, you can create a daily routine that actively supports inflammation reduction. The next chapter of the book will focus on adopting a holistic approach to life, exploring how all these practices combine to form a sustainable health path and lasting well-being.

Chapter 7: Integration And Supplementation

7.1 Embracing a Holistic Approach to Life for Health and Well-being

Section 7.1 of the book emphasizes the importance of embracing a holistic approach to life to promote long-term health and well-being. This perspective integrates not just an anti-inflammatory diet and lifestyle but also a positive mental and emotional attitude. This section prepares the reader for the next section, which will explore the power of an integrated approach that considers the mind, body, and spirit.

Understanding Holism

- **Definition of Holism:** A holistic approach to health considers the person as a whole, encompassing physical, mental, emotional, and spiritual aspects.

- **Interconnection between Life Aspects:** Recognizing that all aspects of life are interconnected and that health in one area affects the others.

Nutrition as Foundation

- **Anti-Inflammatory Diet as Baseline:** The anti-inflammatory diet is crucial but is just one part of the equation. Adequate nutrition supports both physical and mental well-being.

Importance of Physical Exercise

- **Regular Physical Activity:** Exercise is not just for the body but also for the mind. It helps reduce stress, improve mood, and boost self-confidence.

Mental and Emotional Health

- **Stress Management:** Stress management techniques such as meditation, mindfulness, and spending time in nature are crucial.

- **Social Connections:** Maintaining positive relationships and a sense of community contributes to emotional and mental well-being.

Spiritual and Personal Growth

- **Search for Meaning:** Exploring activities that give life meaning and purpose, which can range from spiritual practices to hobbies and volunteering.

- **Self-awareness and Reflection:** Dedicating time to self-awareness and personal reflection can help better understand oneself and find balance in life.

Environment and Lifestyle

- **Healthy Environment:** Creating a home and work environment that supports health and well-being, reducing exposure to toxins and harmful chemicals.

- **Healthy Daily Routines:** Establishing daily routines that promote well-being, such as getting enough sleep, eating at regular times, and allocating time for relaxation.

Transition to the Next Section

After understanding the importance of a holistic approach to life, the next section will specifically explore how to integrate all these elements into a coherent and actionable plan. We will discuss how to balance different aspects of life to support optimal health and lasting well-being.

7.2 Integrating a Holistic Approach into Daily Life

Section 7.2 focuses on the practical integration of a holistic approach to life into the daily routine. This section provides tips on balancing diet, physical exercise, mental health, and activities that nourish the spirit, preparing the reader for the next section that will discuss the importance of regularly evaluating progress and adjusting the approach based on outcomes.

Creating Balance in Daily Life

- **Balanced Planning:** Organize your day to include time for work, relaxation, physical exercise, and personal activities. Avoid overloading your schedule with commitments.

Nutrition and Physical Exercise

- **Regular, Nutritious Meals:** Maintain a regimen of regular meals that include a variety of anti-inflammatory foods.

- **Customized Exercise Routine:** Choose forms of exercise that fit personal preferences and fitness levels, making it easier to maintain them as part of the daily routine.

Stress Management and Mental Health

- **Daily Relaxation Techniques:** Practice relaxation techniques such as meditation or deep breathing every day.

- **Recreational Activities:** Include activities that relax and cheer, such as spending time with friends, reading, listening to music, or pursuing a hobby.

Personal and Spiritual Growth

- **Reflection and Self-awareness:** Dedicate time for personal reflection, which can include journaling, meditating, or participating in personal growth groups.
- **Connectivity and Belonging:** Engage in communities or groups that share similar values and interests, which can be spiritual, cultural, or based on common interests.

Healthy Environment

- **Living and Working Environment:** Create a home and work environment that promotes well-being, such as keeping spaces tidy, increasing natural light, and reducing noise.

- **Connection with Nature:** Spend time outdoors regularly, which can include gardening, nature walks, or simply time spent in a park.

Evaluation and Adaptation

- **Monitoring Progress:** Regularly assess your well-being and progress toward health goals.

- **Flexibility and Adaptation:** Be willing to adjust your routine and habits based on evolving needs and feedback from your body and mind.

Transition to the Next Section

After examining how to integrate a holistic approach into daily life, the next section of the book will explore the importance of regular progress evaluation. We will discuss how consistent monitoring and adjusting strategies can support continuous improvement in health and well-being.

7.3 Regular Evaluation and Path Adjustment

Section 7.3 addresses the importance of regular evaluation and adjustment of the anti-inflammatory path. This section focuses on how to monitor progress and make appropriate changes to continuously improve health and well-being. This approach prepares the reader for the next section, which will discuss how to maintain motivation and long-term commitment.

Monitoring Progress

- **Health Journal:** Keep a journal to record diet, physical activity, stress and sleep levels, helping to identify patterns or areas needing improvement.

- **Regular Self-Assessment:** Conduct regular self-assessments of physical and emotional well-being, noting any changes in symptoms or energy levels.

Using Feedback for Adjustments

- **Body Feedback:** Pay attention to signals from your body, such as improvements or deteriorations in symptoms, and adjust the diet or exercise routine accordingly.

- **Emotional and Mental Feedback:** Acknowledge and respond to signs of stress, anxiety, or mental fatigue, adjusting relaxation techniques or seeking support when necessary.

Engaging Health Professionals

- **Regular Check-Ups:** Undergo regular medical check-ups to monitor parameters like cholesterol levels, blood pressure, and inflammatory markers.

- **Nutritional Counseling:** Work with a dietitian or nutritionist to refine the anti-inflammatory eating plan.

Adjusting Routine Based on Circumstances

- **Life Changes:** Be ready to modify the routine in response to life changes, such as a new job, a health condition, or changes in family life.

- **Flexibility in Practices:** Maintain a flexible approach, adjusting exercises, relaxation practices, or eating habits based on current needs.

Continuous Learning

- **Ongoing Education:** Stay informed about new research and trends in the field of anti-inflammatory nutrition and holistic health.

- **Trying New Techniques:** Be open to trying new methods or practices that may further improve health and well-being.

Transition to the Next Section

After understanding the importance of regularly evaluating and adjusting one's anti-inflammatory journey, the next section will focus on maintaining motivation and long-term commitment. This includes strategies for staying focused on health and well-being goals, despite challenges and obstacles.

7.4 Maintaining Motivation and Long-Term Commitment

Section 7.4 explores strategies for maintaining motivation and long-term commitment to an anti-inflammatory lifestyle. This is crucial to ensure that positive changes introduced become a permanent part of daily life. This section prepares the reader for the next section, which will address how to tackle and overcome obstacles and challenges that may be encountered along the way.

Setting Realistic and Measurable Goals

- **SMART Goals:** Set goals that are Specific, Measurable, Achievable, Relevant, and Time-bound.

- **Small Steps:** Break down long-term goals into smaller, manageable milestones to avoid feeling overwhelmed.

Celebrating Success

- **Acknowledging Progress:** Celebrate small successes along the way, such as improvements in symptoms, increased energy, or reaching exercise milestones.

- **Self-Reward:** Find ways to reward yourself that aren't food-related, like a new book, a massage, or a recreational activity.

Building a Support Network

- **Engaging Family and Friends:** Sharing your goals and plans with family and friends can provide valuable support and encouragement.

- **Support Groups:** Join support groups or online communities where you can share experiences, challenges, and successes.

Maintaining Flexibility

- **Adapting to Changes:** Be ready to modify your plan if circumstances change, maintaining a flexible approach.

- **Learning from Experience:** Use any setbacks or challenges as learning opportunities to strengthen and improve your approach.

Maintaining Awareness and Reflection

- **Regular Self-Reflection:** Dedicate time to personal reflection to assess feelings and thoughts in relation to your journey.

- **Health and Well-being Journal:** Keeping a journal can help track progress and reflect on experiences.

Visualization Techniques and Positive Affirmations

- **Visualization:** Using visualization to imagine success and desired outcomes can be a powerful motivational tool.

- **Positive Affirmations:** Repeating positive affirmations can help maintain a positive and goal-oriented mindset.

Transition to the Next Section

After examining how to maintain motivation and commitment, the next section of the book will address strategies for tackling and overcoming obstacles and challenges that may be encountered on the path to a holistic approach to health.

7.5 Tackling and Overcoming Obstacles and Challenges

Section 7.5 focuses on how to tackle and overcome obstacles and challenges that may arise on the journey towards an anti-inflammatory lifestyle. This section provides strategies for dealing with common difficulties, preparing the reader for the next chapter, which will introduce the concept of resilience and adaptability in the context of an anti-inflammatory life.

Acknowledging and Accepting Obstacles

- **Identifying Challenges:** Identify both internal and external obstacles that can interfere with the anti-inflammatory path.

- **Acceptance:** Accept that challenges are part of the process and do not signify failure.

Strategies to Overcome Difficulties

- **Flexible Thinking:** Adopt a flexible mental approach, ready to change strategies when circumstances shift.

- **Seeking Alternative Solutions:** Be creative in finding alternative solutions when one strategy doesn't work.

Managing Relapses or Setbacks

- **Non-Punitive Approach:** Treat any relapses or setbacks as learning opportunities rather than sources of self-criticism.

- **Action Plan for Relapses:** Having a clear action plan for when setbacks occur can help quickly get back on track.

Sustaining Motivation

- **Remembering the 'Why':** Keeping a clear understanding of why you chose an anti-inflammatory path can help stay motivated in the face of challenges.

- **Visualizing the Benefits:** Focus on the long-term benefits of the anti-inflammatory diet and lifestyle to maintain inspiration.

Seeking and Receiving Support

- **Asking for Help:** Don't hesitate to seek help from health professionals, friends, or support groups when needed.

- **Sharing Experiences:** Sharing experiences, challenges, and successes with others can provide support and new perspectives.

Promoting Resilience

- **Building Resilience:** Develop resilience through regular practice of stress management, physical activity, and relaxation techniques.

- **Appreciating Small Successes:** Celebrate small advancements and recognize your own strength in overcoming difficulties.

Transition to the Next Section

After discussing strategies for tackling obstacles and challenges, the next chapter will focus on building resilience and adaptability, key elements for long-term success in a holistic approach to anti-inflammatory health.

Chapter 8: Addressing Common Challenges and Obstacles

8.1 Building Resilience and Adaptability

Section 8.1 of the book is dedicated to building resilience and adaptability, essential qualities for maintaining a long-term anti-inflammatory lifestyle. This section offers insights and strategies on how to develop and strengthen these qualities, serving as an introduction to the next section, which will discuss the importance of continuous self-improvement and learning.

Concepts of Resilience and Adaptability

- **Definition of Resilience:** Resilience is the ability to bounce back from adversity, maintaining a positive and proactive attitude.

- **Importance of Adaptability:** Adaptability refers to the ability to change one's approach and behavior in response to changes and challenges.

Developing Resilience

- **Positive Mindset:** Cultivate a positive attitude towards challenges, seeing them as opportunities for growth rather than insurmountable obstacles.

- **Stress Management Techniques:** Regularly practice stress management techniques, such as meditation, yoga, and physical exercise, to improve the ability to effectively handle stressful situations.

Encouraging Adaptability

- **Flexibility in Thinking and Behavior:** Be open to changing the way you think and act in the face of new information or situations.

- **Experimentation and Learning:** Try new approaches and strategies, accepting that the learning process may include mistakes and revisions.

Building a Support Network

- **Supportive Relationships:** Maintain and develop relationships with family, friends, and health professionals who can offer support and advice.

- **Communities and Groups:** Participate in groups or communities that share similar interests or lifestyles, to exchange ideas and experiences.

Managing Emotions

- **Recognizing Emotions:** Learn to recognize and accept your emotions, rather than avoiding or suppressing them.

- **Emotional Processing Techniques:** Use techniques such as writing, art, or therapy to process and understand emotions.

Increasing Knowledge and Skills

- **Continuous Learning:** Engage in continuous learning about health, diet, and overall well-being.

- **Personal Development:** Attend seminars, workshops, or read books that contribute to personal growth and the expansion of your skills.

Transition to the Next Section

After exploring how to build resilience and adaptability, the next section will address the importance of continuous self-improvement and learning. We will discuss how constant commitment to self-development can enrich and further strengthen the anti-inflammatory journey.

8.2 Continuous Self-Improvement and Learning

Section 8.2 of the book focuses on continuous self-improvement and learning as key elements to maintaining and enhancing an anti-inflammatory lifestyle over time. This section emphasizes the importance of ongoing learning and personal evolution, setting the stage for the next section, which will discuss adapting the anti-inflammatory diet and lifestyle to different life stages.

Meaning of Continuous Self-Improvement

- **Personal Growth:** Acknowledge that the journey towards health and wellness is an ongoing process that requires commitment and dedication.

- **Growth Mindset:** Develop a growth mindset, be open to new ideas, and willing to change habits as necessary.

Strategies for Ongoing Learning

- **Formal and Informal Education:** Engage in courses, seminars, workshops, or conferences focusing on health, nutrition, stress management, and overall well-being.

- **Reading and Research:** Stay updated with the latest literature on anti-inflammatory diet, physical exercise, mental health, and holistic wellness.

Experimentation and Adaptation

- **Trial and Error:** Be willing to experiment with different techniques, foods, and activities to find out what works best for your health and wellness.

- **Adapting to Body's Responses:** Listen closely to your body and make adjustments based on how it reacts to different foods, exercises, and stress management practices.

Reflection and Self-Awareness

- **Personal Journal:** Keep a personal journal to reflect on experiences, feelings, and progress.

- **Meditation and Mindfulness:** Practice meditation and mindfulness to develop greater self-awareness and better understand your needs and reactions.

Building Community and Sharing Knowledge

- **Community Participation:** Get involved in online or local communities that share similar interests to exchange knowledge, experiences, and support.

- **Mentorship and Coaching:** Consider working with a coach or mentor for personalized guidance and support.

Transition to the Next Section

After discussing the importance of self-improvement and ongoing learning, the next section will explore how to adapt the anti-inflammatory diet and lifestyle to different life stages. This includes adjustments to changes such as aging, hormonal shifts, activity levels, and other life circumstances.

8.3 Adapting Diet and Lifestyle to Different Life Stages

Section 8.3 of the book focuses on adapting the anti-inflammatory diet and lifestyle to different life stages. This section explores how the body's needs change with age, hormonal shifts, activity levels, and other life circumstances, setting the stage for the next section, which will discuss the importance of integrating and balancing the nutritional, physical, and mental aspects of the anti-inflammatory lifestyle.

Understanding Different Life Stages

- **Physiological Variations:** Acknowledge that the body undergoes natural changes throughout life, which can affect nutritional and exercise needs.

- **Adapting to Evolving Needs:** Be ready to modify diet and exercise routines in response to these changes.

Diet and Lifestyle at Different Ages

- **Young Adults:** Focus on a balanced, nutrient-rich diet to support active growth and development.

- **Adulthood:** Maintain a balance of macronutrients, monitor calorie intake, and incorporate regular exercise to manage weight and prevent chronic diseases.

- **Seniors:** Increase intake of calcium and vitamin D to support bone health, and adapt exercise to maintain muscle strength and balance.

Hormonal Changes and Reproductive Health

- **Pregnancy and Breastfeeding:** Increase intake of specific nutrients such as folic acid, iron, and calcium.

- **Menopause and Andropause:** Adapt diet to address hormonal changes, focus on foods rich in phytoestrogens, and manage metabolic shifts.

Adapting to Lifestyle Changes

- **Work Routine Changes:** Modify diet and exercise routine in response to changes in work routine, such as shifting from a physically active job to a sedentary one.

- **Periods of Stress or Illness:** Increase intake of nutrient-rich foods and potentially supplement with vitamins and minerals during periods of stress or illness.

Regular Monitoring and Evaluation

- **Regular Medical Checkups:** Undergo regular medical examinations to monitor health and receive personalized advice on diet and exercise.

- **Self-Assessment:** Be attentive to your body's signals and make adjustments when changes in health or well-being are perceived.

Transition to the Next Section

After exploring how to adapt the anti-inflammatory diet and lifestyle to different life stages, the next section of the book will focus on integrating and balancing the nutritional, physical, and mental aspects for a holistic and sustainable approach to the anti-inflammatory lifestyle.

8.4 Integrating and Balancing Nutritional, Physical, and Mental Aspects

Section 8.4 of the book is dedicated to the integration and balance of nutritional, physical, and mental aspects within the anti-inflammatory lifestyle. This holistic approach is essential for maximizing overall health benefits and well-being. This section prepares the reader for the next point, discussing the importance of consistency and a daily routine in adopting a sustainable anti-inflammatory lifestyle.

The Importance of a Holistic Approach

- **Interconnectedness of Body, Mind, and Spirit:** Acknowledge that physical, mental, and spiritual health are deeply interconnected, and well-being in one area affects the others.

- **Integrated Approach:** Adopt an approach that simultaneously considers diet, physical activity, and mental health.

Holistic Nutrition

- **Balanced Diet:** Ensure the diet includes a variety of anti-inflammatory foods, balancing both macro and micronutrients.

- **Listen to Your Body:** Be attentive to your body's signals and adjust food intake based on personal needs.

Balanced Physical Activity

- **Regular Exercise:** Integrate various forms of physical exercise, from aerobic activities to strength and flexibility exercises, for a balanced approach.

- **Body Listening:** Modify the intensity and type of exercise based on physical conditions and energy levels.

Mental and Emotional Health

- **Stress Management:** Incorporate regular stress management practices such as meditation, yoga, and deep breathing.

- **Time for Relaxation and Rest:** Ensure there's time for relaxation and rest, allowing the body and mind to recover.

Personal and Spiritual Growth

- **Personal Reflection:** Dedicate time to personal reflection to foster inner growth and self-understanding.

- **Spirit-Enriching Activities:** Engage in activities that nourish the spirit, such as volunteering, art, or connecting with nature.

Balancing Daily Life

- **Work-Life Balance:** Maintain a healthy balance between work and leisure to prevent burnout and excessive stress.

- **Healthy Daily Routines:** Establish daily routines that support all aspects of health and well-being.

Transition to the Next Point

After exploring the integration and balance of nutrition, physical exercise, and mental health, the next point of the book will discuss the importance of maintaining consistency and establishing an effective daily routine in adopting a sustainable anti-inflammatory lifestyle.

8.5 Maintaining Consistency and Establishing a Daily Routine

Section 8.5 addresses the importance of maintaining consistency and establishing a daily routine when adopting an anti-inflammatory lifestyle. This is essential to ensure that changes are sustainable and lead to long-term benefits. This section prepares the reader for the final chapter, which will cover the long-term vision and continuous adaptation of an anti-inflammatory lifestyle.

Creating Sustainable Habits

- **Daily Routines:** Develop daily routines that include anti-inflammatory eating, physical exercise, and stress management.

- **Progressive Small Changes:** Start with small changes and gradually build upon them, making long-term adherence easier.

Consistency in Diet

- **Meal Planning:** Plan meals in advance to avoid impulsive food decisions that may deviate from an anti-inflammatory diet.

- **Meal Preparation:** Dedicating time to meal prep can help maintain a healthy and balanced diet.

Regular Exercise Routine

- **Exercise Planning:** Establish a regular exercise schedule, considering the time, type, and intensity of physical activity.

- **Physical Activity Integrated into Daily Life:** Find ways to incorporate more movement into everyday life, like walking more or using the stairs.

Daily Stress Management

- **Relaxation Practices:** Incorporate relaxation practices such as meditation, deep breathing, or yoga into the daily routine.

- **Break Moments:** Take short breaks throughout the day to reduce stress and recharge.

Monitoring and Self-Assessment

- **Health and Wellness Journal:** Keep a journal to track diet, exercise, and stress levels, helping to identify areas needing improvement.

- **Regular Reflection and Assessment:** Dedicate time to reflect on progress and evaluate what works well and what could be improved.

Sustaining Motivation

- **Short and Long-Term Goals:** Set clear and achievable goals to keep motivation high.

- **Celebrating Successes:** Recognize and celebrate milestones to maintain enthusiasm and motivation.

Transition to the Next Chapter

Having established the importance of maintaining consistency and a daily routine, the next chapter of the book will explore the long-term vision of an anti-inflammatory lifestyle. We will discuss how to continue adapting and evolving, keeping the lifestyle aligned with life changes and personal needs.

Chapter 9: Success Stories and Case Studies

9.1 Long-Term Vision for an Anti-Inflammatory Lifestyle

Section 9.1 of the book explores the long-term vision of an anti-inflammatory lifestyle. This chapter emphasizes the importance of looking beyond short-term changes, focusing on how an anti-inflammatory approach can evolve and adapt over a lifetime. This section prepares the reader for the next point, which will discuss how to face life's inevitable changes and maintain a flexible anti-inflammatory approach.

Understanding the Evolving Nature of the Anti-Inflammatory Lifestyle

- **Continuous Adaptation:** Acknowledge that an anti-inflammatory lifestyle may require adjustments as personal needs, health conditions, and life stages change.

- **Learning from Experience:** Use past experiences as learning opportunities to refine and improve the approach over time.

Long-Term Sustainability

- **Lasting Lifestyle Choices:** Focus on lifestyle choices that are sustainable in the long term rather than quick fixes.

- **Balance and Moderation:** Find a balance between strict diet adherence and flexibility to enjoy life while maintaining health and well-being.

Incorporating New Research and Information

- **Continuous Updating:** Stay informed about the latest research in nutrition and health to integrate new information and approaches into one's lifestyle.

- **Ongoing Education:** Engage in courses, seminars, and workshops to expand understanding and skills related to health and wellness.

Long-Term Planning

- **Personalized Health Plans:** Develop health plans that consider long-term goals, such as disease prevention or maintaining mobility and energy.

- **Collaboration with Health Professionals:** Work with doctors, nutritionists, and other health experts to monitor health and adapt the anti-inflammatory life plan.

Maintaining Flexibility and Resilience

- **Readiness for Changes:** Be ready to adapt to life changes, both expected and unexpected, maintaining a flexible mindset.

- **Resilience in the Face of Challenges:** Cultivate resilience to face challenges and obstacles that arise along the way.

Transition to the Next Point

Having outlined the importance of a long-term vision for an anti-inflammatory lifestyle, the next point of the book will focus on how to face life changes, whether related to age, work, family, or other circumstances, and how to maintain a flexible and effective anti-inflammatory lifestyle through these changes.

9.2 Navigating Life Changes with a Flexible Anti-Inflammatory Approach

Chapter 9.2 focuses on how to navigate life changes while maintaining a flexible and effective anti-inflammatory approach. This chapter provides strategies for adapting the anti-inflammatory lifestyle to various situations and life stages, preparing the reader for the next point, which will explore how to consciously integrate these practices into a harmonious and balanced life journey.

Adapting to Significant Changes

- **Transition Phases:** Whether it's a job change, a new family phase, or moving homes, acknowledge that these transitions may require adjustments in the anti-inflammatory lifestyle.

- **Flexibility in Meal and Exercise Planning:** Modify meal planning and physical activity to fit new schedules and routines.

Managing Dietary Changes

- **Eating in Different Situations:** Adapt food choices in situations like travel, holidays, or social events to maintain the anti-inflammatory approach while enjoying new experiences.

- **Flexible Food Options:** Explore diverse culinary options that fit the anti-inflammatory lifestyle, even when dining out or traveling.

Addressing Physical Health Changes

- **Adjusting Physical Exercise:** Modify the exercise regime in response to changes in physical health, such as injuries or emerging medical conditions.

- **Dialogue with Health Professionals:** Regularly consult health professionals to adapt diet and exercise to evolving health needs.

Emotional Response to Changes

- **Emotional Support:** Seek emotional support during times of significant change to maintain mental balance and keep stress in check.

- **Stress Management Techniques:** Continue to use stress management techniques such as meditation, yoga, and mindful breathing during periods of change.

Maintaining Awareness and Balance

- **Self-Reflection:** Dedicate regular time to self-reflection to assess how changes are affecting overall well-being.

- **Balancing Various Life Aspects:** Strive to maintain a balance between work, family life, leisure, and self-care.

Transition to the Next Point

After examining how to navigate life changes while maintaining a flexible anti-inflammatory approach, the next point will explore how to consciously integrate these practices into a harmonious and balanced life journey, emphasizing the importance of a holistic and long-lasting approach to well-being.

9.3 Consciously Integrating Anti-Inflammatory Practices into a Harmonious Life Path

This section delves into how to consciously incorporate anti-inflammatory practices into a balanced and harmonious life journey. It emphasizes the importance of a holistic approach that balances diet, physical activity, mental health, and emotional well-being, setting the stage for the next point, which will discuss maintaining this lifestyle within the context of social relationships and interactions.

Creating a Holistic Balance

- **Holistic Well-being:** Understanding that health is not just the absence of disease but a harmonious balance between physical, mental, emotional, and social well-being.

- **Integrated Approach:** Adopting an integrated approach that includes anti-inflammatory nutrition, regular physical activity, stress management, and time for activities that enrich the spirit.

Mindful Eating

- **Intentional Eating:** Choosing foods not only for their anti-inflammatory benefits but also for the pleasure and satisfaction they bring.

- **Listening to the Body:** Being attentive to the body's signals and choosing foods that support individual well-being.

Balanced Physical Activity

- **Exercise Variety:** Varying exercise routines to include aerobic activities, strength training, flexibility exercises, and relaxation practices.

- **Listening and Respecting Physical Limits:** Acknowledging and respecting the body's limits, avoiding overexertion and injury.

Stress Management and Mental Health

- **Daily Relaxation Practices:** Incorporating daily practices such as meditation, mindful breathing, and spending time in nature.

- **Moments of Quietude:** Allocating time for moments of quiet and solitude to foster mental rest and renewal.

Spiritual and Personal Growth

- **Reflection and Personal Growth:** Dedicating time to personal reflection, volunteering, or hobbies that nourish the spirit and sense of fulfillment.

- **Deep Connections:** Cultivating deep and meaningful relationships that support emotional and spiritual well-being.

Adapting to Life's Rhythms

- **Flexibility and Adaptability:** Being flexible and adaptable to different life stages and challenges, maintaining a balance across various aspects of life.

- **Consistency and Persistence:** Keeping a steady course in anti-inflammatory practices while adapting them to changing needs over time.

Transition to the Next Point

After considering how to consciously integrate anti-inflammatory practices into a harmonious life balance, the next point will examine how to maintain this lifestyle within the context of social relationships and interactions, highlighting the importance of a supportive community and healthy relationships.

9.4 Maintaining an Anti-Inflammatory Lifestyle in Social Relationships

This section delves into how to sustain an anti-inflammatory lifestyle amidst social relationships, underscoring the significance of forging and upholding a social network that supports and enriches this journey. It sets the stage for the following discussion on the role of community and social support in fostering and maintaining an anti-inflammatory lifestyle.

Importance of Social Relationships

- **Support and Understanding:** Having a support network that comprehends and respects the choice of an anti-inflammatory lifestyle.

- **Effective Communication:** Mastering the art of communicating one's lifestyle choices and needs regarding the anti-inflammatory lifestyle to friends and family.

Navigating Social Situations

- **Restaurants and Social Gatherings:** Developing strategies for making healthy food choices when dining out or attending social events.

- **Flexibility and Balance:** Finding a balance between adhering to the diet and enjoying social interactions, without feeling isolated or restricted.

Encouragement and Role Modeling

- **Being a Positive Role Model:** Acting as a positive exemplar for others, demonstrating how an anti-inflammatory lifestyle can be both healthy and enjoyable.

- **Mutual Encouragement:** Creating an environment where friends and family encourage each other in pursuing healthy lifestyle choices.

Building Supportive Communities

- **Groups and Communities:** Joining or forming groups and communities, both online and offline, that share an interest in an anti-inflammatory lifestyle.

- **Participation in Events:** Engaging in events, seminars, and workshops related to the anti-inflammatory lifestyle to connect with like-minded individuals.

Managing Conflicts and Differences

- **Respecting Differences:** Honoring others' lifestyle choices and expecting the same respect in return.

- **Navigating Disagreements:** Learning to handle disagreements or misunderstandings about lifestyle choices constructively.

Positive Influence and Inspiration

- **Sharing Experiences and Knowledge:** Sharing one's experiences and insights on the anti-inflammatory lifestyle, inspiring others to consider healthier life choices.

- **Listening and Empathy:** Being attentive listeners and showing empathy in interactions, fostering an environment of mutual support.

Transition to the Next Point

After examining the importance of social relationships in an anti-inflammatory lifestyle, the next section of the book will focus on the role of community and social support. We will discuss how community can play a crucial role in supporting, motivating, and enriching the journey toward anti-inflammatory well-being.

9.5 The Role of Community and Social Support

This section focuses on the pivotal role of community and social support in fostering and maintaining an anti-inflammatory lifestyle. It explores how a social network can provide support, inspiration, and resources for those on an anti-inflammatory journey. This chapter sets the stage for the final chapter, emphasizing the importance of a holistic approach and providing a general conclusion for the book.

Importance of Social Support

- **Emotional and Practical Support:** Understanding how a support network can offer crucial emotional and practical assistance in maintaining a healthy lifestyle.

- **Sharing Experiences:** Sharing experiences with others can provide valuable advice, coping strategies, and a sense of camaraderie on the journey.

Creating or Finding Support Communities

- **Local and Online Groups:** Participating in or forming support groups, both locally and online, where ideas, recipes, successes, and challenges can be shared.

- **Workshops and Seminars:** Attending educational events and workshops can be an excellent way to learn and connect with others sharing similar goals.

Role of Family and Friendship Relationships

- **Engaging Family and Friends:** Informing family and friends about one's lifestyle and its importance, seeking their support and understanding.

- **Shared Social Activities:** Organizing or participating in social activities aligned with the anti-inflammatory lifestyle, such as cooking groups or walking clubs.

Professional Support

- **Consulting Experts:** Seeking support from health professionals, like nutritionists, therapists, or health coaches, who can offer specific advice and personalized support.

- **Professional Health Networks:** Utilizing professional networks to stay informed about new research and trends in anti-inflammatory health.

Benefits of Community

- **Motivation and Inspiration:** Receiving motivation and inspiration from others can help stay focused and committed to the journey.

- **Learning Through Sharing:** Learning from others through the sharing of success stories, practical advice, and solutions to common challenges.

Transition to the Next Chapter

Concluding the discussion on the role of community and social support, the next chapter will recap the main themes of the book, emphasizing the importance of a holistic approach to the anti-inflammatory lifestyle and providing a general conclusion and reflection on the journey undertaken.

Chapter 10: Conclusion And Next Steps

10.1 Conclusions and Reflections on the Anti-Inflammatory Journey

This section of the book provides an overall reflection on the journey towards an anti-inflammatory lifestyle, summarizing key concepts and highlights from the previous chapters. This conclusion offers a general overview and reflection on the undertaken journey, preparing the reader for the next section, which will provide final advice and tips for maintaining commitment and motivation over time.

Summary of Key Principles

- **Importance of an Anti-Inflammatory Diet:** Recapitulating how a diet rich in anti-inflammatory foods can positively impact health and reduce the risk of chronic diseases.

- **Role of Physical Exercise and Stress Management:** Emphasizing the significance of regular physical activity and stress management techniques for overall well-being.

Lessons Learned and Personal Growth

- **Development of Awareness and Resilience:** Reflecting on how the anti-inflammatory journey may have enhanced personal awareness, resilience, and adaptability.

- **Key Learnings:** Reviewing key learnings from the journey, including self-improvement, adaptability, and the importance of social support.

Reflection on the Holistic Approach

- **Balancing Body, Mind, and Spirit:** Reflecting on how the holistic approach has positively influenced not only physical health but also mental and emotional well-being.

- **Integration into Daily Life:** Discussing how integrating anti-inflammatory practices into daily life can lead to more comprehensive and lasting well-being.

Challenges and Obstacles Overcome

- **Acknowledgment of Challenges:** Recognizing the obstacles faced along the way and how they were overcome.
- **Growth Through Challenges:** Understanding how overcoming these challenges has contributed to personal growth and the maturation of the anti-inflammatory approach.

Future Vision and Maintenance

- **Looking Forward:** Considering how to continue maintaining and adapting the anti-inflammatory lifestyle in the face of future life changes.
- **Long-Term Maintenance:** Emphasizing the importance of ongoing self-improvement and maintaining anti-inflammatory practices.

Transition to the Next Section

Concluding this chapter of reflection and summary, the next section will provide final advice and strategies to support the commitment and motivation in maintaining an anti-inflammatory lifestyle in the long term, ensuring that the benefits achieved can be preserved and expanded over time.

10.2 Final Advice for Long-Term Maintenance

This section of the book provides final advice and strategies to support commitment and motivation in the long-term maintenance of an anti-inflammatory lifestyle. This chapter aims to equip the reader with practical tools and tips to ensure that the healthy habits developed can continue to thrive. This section sets the stage for the next point, which will explore the theme of continuous evolution and customization of the anti-inflammatory lifestyle.

Strengthening Commitment

- **Remember the 'Why':** Always keep in mind the personal reason that motivated the adoption of an anti-inflammatory lifestyle, which can serve as a powerful motivator.

- **Acknowledgment of Benefits:** Continue to acknowledge and celebrate the benefits this lifestyle brings to health and overall well-being.

Strategies for Sustainability

- **Planning and Organization:** Continue planning meals and exercises in advance to avoid impulsive decisions and maintain consistency.

- **Flexibility and Adaptability:** Be ready to adapt the diet and exercise routine in response to changes in personal and professional life.

Building a Support Community

- **Sharing and Connection:** Maintain and strengthen relationships with people who support or share an anti-inflammatory lifestyle.

- **Participation in Groups and Forums:** Active participation in related groups and forums remains important for sharing experiences and receiving support.

Self-Evaluation and Monitoring

- **Regular Assessments:** Conduct regular self-assessments to monitor physical and mental health and make any necessary adjustments.

- **Use of Diaries and Apps:** Use diaries, apps, or other tools to track diet, exercise, and stress levels.

Continuous Learning

- **Updating and Education:** Stay informed about the latest research and trends in the field of anti-inflammatory health and wellness.

- **Exploration of New Practices:** Experiment with new stress management techniques, new foods, or forms of exercise to keep the experience alive.

Maintaining Balance in Daily Life

- **Work-Life Balance:** Continue to work towards a balance between work, leisure, family, and self-care.

- **Time for Rest and Relaxation:** Ensure there is enough time for rest and activities that relax and enrich the mind and spirit.

Transition to the Next Point

With these final tips for long-term maintenance, the next point will explore the concept of continuous evolution and personalization of the anti-inflammatory lifestyle. We will discuss how the journey towards wellness is an ongoing process, requiring personalized adaptations to meet changing individual needs over time.

10.3 Continuous Evolution and Personalization of the Anti-Inflammatory Lifestyle

This section addresses the importance of continuous evolution and personalization in the anti-inflammatory lifestyle. It emphasizes how individual needs change over time and how essential it is to adapt and refine the approach to stay aligned with these variations. The reader is prepared for the next point, which will discuss the role of innovation and experimentation in adopting an anti-inflammatory lifestyle.

Adaptability to Life Changes

- **Responding to Physical Changes:** Adapt diet and exercise in response to changes such as aging, pregnancy, or hormonal shifts.

- **Listening to Your Body:** Stay tuned to your body, recognizing and responding to its signals to optimize health and well-being.

Personalization of Approach

- **Customized Diet:** Personalize the diet based on individual preferences, food tolerances, and specific health goals.

- **Tailored Exercise:** Choose forms of exercise that fit one's fitness level, interests, and personal lifestyle.

Personal Growth and Development

- **Self-Awareness:** Continue to develop self-awareness through reflection and self-assessment, understanding one's needs and preferences better.

- **Continuous Learning:** Maintain a mindset of continuous learning, exploring new research and approaches in the field of anti-inflammatory health.

Adaptation to Modern Life

- **Innovation and Technology:** Utilize technology and innovation to support the anti-inflammatory lifestyle, such as health tracking apps or online recipes.

- **Balancing with Modern Life:** Find a balance between maintaining anti-inflammatory practices and the demands of a modern, busy life.

Sharing and Communication

- **Sharing Experiences:** Share your experiences and what you've learned with others, contributing to the community and learning from others.

- **Open Communication with Health Professionals:** Regularly dialogue with health professionals to receive advice and adjust the health plan based on feedback.

Transition to the Next Point

Concluding the discussion on evolution and personalization of the anti-inflammatory lifestyle, the next point will explore the importance of innovation and experimentation. This will include exploring new foods, exercise practices, and stress management techniques, as well as staying open to new research and emerging approaches in the field of anti-inflammatory health.

10.4 Innovation and Experimentation in the Anti-Inflammatory Journey

This section of the book delves into the importance of innovation and experimentation in maintaining an anti-inflammatory lifestyle. It encourages readers to remain open and creative when exploring new foods, exercise practices, and stress management techniques, preparing them for the next section that will offer a final reflection and advice for continuing the wellness journey.

Exploring New Foods and Recipes

- **Culinary Experimentation:** Encourage the exploration of new foods and recipes that align with an anti-inflammatory diet.

- **Creativity in Cooking:** Use the kitchen as a space for creativity, experimenting with different ingredients and cooking techniques to keep the diet exciting and varied.

Innovation in Physical Exercise

- **Trying New Activities:** Be open to trying new forms of physical activity that can be fun, challenging, and beneficial.

- **Integrating Technologies:** Leverage emerging technologies, such as fitness apps or wearable devices, to enhance and diversify the exercise routine.

Advanced Stress Management Techniques

- **Modern Approaches to Stress Reduction:** Explore new techniques for stress management, like virtual reality, guided meditation, or innovative relaxation therapies.

- **Customizing Relaxation Practices:** Tailor relaxation techniques to individual preferences and life circumstance changes.

Maintaining Openness and Curiosity

- **Continuous Learning:** Always be open to new information and research in the field of anti-inflammatory health.

- **Stay Curious and Experiment:** Maintain a curious mindset, experimenting with and adapting new ideas and approaches.

Collaboration and Knowledge Sharing

- **Collaborating with Others:** Share discoveries and experiences with the community, learning from others' successes and challenges.

- **Participating in Online and Offline Communities:** Stay active in both online and offline communities to stay informed about the latest trends and innovations.

Transition to the Next Section

After exploring the importance of innovation and experimentation, the next section will offer a final reflection on the journey towards an anti-inflammatory lifestyle. It will provide advice and inspiration for continuing to grow and evolve on the path of wellness.

10.5 Final Reflection and Continuing the Wellness Journey

This section concludes the book with a final reflection, offering a perspective for the future and encouraging the reader to persist in their journey towards an anti-inflammatory lifestyle. This section aims to consolidate the concepts learned and to motivate the reader to continue on their path with confidence and determination.

Summary of Key Concepts

- **Reflection on Key Learnings:** Reflect on the key concepts learned throughout the book, including the benefits of an anti-inflammatory diet, the importance of physical exercise, stress management, and social support.

- **Value of Holistic Health:** Emphasize the value of a holistic approach to health that integrates body, mind, and spirit.

Importance of Consistency and Change

- **Long-Term Maintenance:** Discuss the importance of maintaining consistency in anti-inflammatory habits while remaining open to change and adaptation.

- **Flexibility and Personal Growth:** Highlight how flexibility and openness to personal growth are essential to navigate effectively on the path of health and wellness.

Inspiration for the Future

- **Long-Term Vision:** Encourage the reader to develop a long-term vision for their health and wellness, looking beyond immediate challenges and focusing on future goals.

- **Power of Personal Example:** Underline how individual choices can inspire and positively influence others.

Strategies to Maintain Motivation

- **Goals and Celebrations:** Suggest setting regular goals and celebrating milestones reached as a means to maintain motivation.

- **Community and Support Network:** Remind the importance of staying connected with a support community for encouragement and inspiration.

With this reflective conclusion, the reader is equipped with the insights and encouragement needed to continue their wellness journey. This final note reiterates the ongoing nature of personal health and wellness endeavors, encouraging continuous engagement, adaptation, and growth.

Chapter 11: Easy and Quick Recipes

Beetroot and Orange Salad with Walnuts

Ingredients:

- 3 medium beetroots, cooked and sliced

- 2 oranges, peeled and sliced

- 1/2 cup of roughly chopped walnuts

- 2 tablespoons of extra virgin olive oil

- 1 tablespoon of balsamic vinegar

- Salt and black pepper, to taste

- 1 tablespoon of honey (optional)

- A pinch of fresh or dried thyme

Nutritional Values (per serving):

- Calories: about 200-250 kcal

- Protein: 3-4 g

- Fats: 15-20 g (mainly monounsaturated and polyunsaturated fats)

- Carbohydrates: 20-25 g

- Fiber: 4-5 g

- Sugars: 12-15 g (naturally from oranges and beetroots)

Preparation:

1. **Prepare the Beetroots:** If you don't have pre-cooked beetroots, boil them in water for about 40-50 minutes or until tender. Let them cool, then peel and slice them.

2. **Prepare the Oranges:** Peel the oranges, removing all the white pith. Slice them into rounds or segments.

3. **Toast the Walnuts:** In a small pan, toast the chopped walnuts over medium heat for 3-5 minutes, until they become slightly golden and aromatic. Let them cool.

4. **Prepare the Vinaigrette:** In a small bowl, mix the olive oil with the balsamic vinegar, a pinch of salt, black pepper, and honey (if using). Add the thyme and mix well.

5. **Assemble the Salad:** Arrange the beetroot and orange slices on a serving plate. Sprinkle the toasted walnuts over the top.

6. **Dress the Salad:** Pour the vinaigrette over the salad just before serving. Adjust salt and pepper, if necessary.

Serve: The salad is now ready to be served. It can be an excellent appetizer or a light and flavorful side dish.

This recipe combines the sweetness of oranges and beetroots with the crunchiness of toasted walnuts, creating a dish rich in flavors and textures, as well as being nutritious and in line with an anti-inflammatory diet.

Cod Fillets with Lemon and Thyme

Ingredients:

- 4 cod fillets (about 150 g each)

- 2 lemons, one juiced and one sliced

- 2 tablespoons of extra virgin olive oil

- 2 cloves of garlic, finely chopped

- 1 tablespoon of fresh thyme (or 1 teaspoon of dried thyme)

- Salt and black pepper, to taste

- Chopped fresh parsley for garnish (optional)

Nutritional Values (per serving):

- Calories: about 200-250 kcal

- Protein: 23-28 g

- Fats: 10-12 g

- Carbohydrates: 3-5 g

- Fiber: 1-2 g

- Sugars: less than 1 g

Preparation:

1. **Prepare the Cod:** Preheat the oven to 200°C (392°F). Lightly grease a baking dish.

2. **Marinate the Cod:** In a bowl, mix the lemon juice, olive oil, chopped garlic, and thyme. Add salt and pepper to taste. Dip the cod fillets in the marinade, ensuring they are completely covered. Let them marinate for about 15-20 minutes.

3. **Cook the Cod:** Place the cod fillets in the baking dish. Pour the rest of the marinade over them. Add lemon slices on top of the fillets.

4. **Bake:** Bake the cod for about 12-15 minutes or until the fish flakes easily with a fork.

5. **Garnish and Serve:** Remove the cod fillets from the oven. Garnish with chopped fresh parsley, if desired. Serve immediately.

This recipe is a great way to enjoy cod, a lean fish rich in protein and omega-3 fatty acids. The lemon and thyme add a fresh and aromatic flavor that enhances the delicacy of the fish.

Broccoli and Kale Soup with Ginger

Ingredients:

- 1 large head of broccoli, cut into florets

- 1/2 green cabbage, chopped

- 1 medium onion, chopped

- 2 cloves of garlic, chopped

- 1 piece of fresh ginger (about 2 cm), grated

- 1 liter of low-sodium vegetable or chicken broth

- 2 tablespoons of extra virgin olive oil

- Salt and black pepper, to taste

- A pinch of chili flakes (optional)

- Juice of 1/2 lemon

Nutritional Values (per serving):

- Calories: about 100-150 kcal

- Protein: 4-6 g

- Fats: 5-7 g

- Carbohydrates: 15-20 g

- Fiber: 5-6 g

- Sugars: 3-4 g

Preparation:

1. **Sauté the Vegetables:** In a large pot, heat the olive oil over medium heat. Add the chopped onion and cook until it becomes translucent, about 5 minutes. Add the garlic and grated ginger, and cook for another 1-2 minutes.

2. **Add Broccoli and Cabbage:** Add the broccoli florets and chopped cabbage. Stir well and cook for about 5 minutes, until the vegetables start to become tender.

3. **Pour in the Broth:** Add the vegetable or chicken broth. Bring to a boil, then reduce the heat and simmer.

4. **Cook the Soup:** Let the soup simmer for about 15-20 minutes or until the vegetables are completely cooked.

5. **Season:** Season with salt and pepper. If you like, add a pinch of chili flakes for a spicy kick. Squeeze the lemon juice into the soup to add freshness.

6. **Blend (Optional):** For a creamier soup, you can blend half of the soup with an immersion blender and then mix it back with the rest.

7. **Serve:** Serve the soup hot. It's great on its own or accompanied by whole-grain croutons.

This soup is rich in nutrients, fiber, and antioxidants, perfect for an anti-inflammatory diet. The combination of broccoli, kale, and ginger offers a powerful anti-inflammatory and detoxifying effect.

Green Smoothie with Spinach, Apple, and Ginger

Ingredients:

- 2 cups of fresh spinach

- 1 large apple, peeled and chopped

- 1 piece of fresh ginger (about 2 cm), peeled and grated

- 1 ripe banana

- 1/2 cup of Greek yogurt or coconut yogurt

- 1 cup of almond milk or other plant-based milk

- 1 tablespoon of chia seeds

- 1 teaspoon of honey or maple syrup (optional)

- Ice (optional)

Nutritional Values (per serving):
- Calories: about 250-300 kcal

- Protein: 8-10 g

- Fats: 5-7 g

- Carbohydrates: 45-50 g

- Fiber: 8-10 g

- Sugars: 20-25 g

Preparation:

1. **Prepare the Ingredients:** Wash the spinach and chop the apple. Peel and grate the ginger. Peel the banana.

2. **Assemble the Smoothie:** Place the spinach, apple, grated ginger, banana, yogurt, almond milk, chia seeds, and sweetener (if using) in the blender.

3. **Blend:** Blend the ingredients on high speed until smooth and creamy. If the smoothie is too thick, add a little more almond milk to reach the desired consistency.

4. **Add Ice (Optional):** If you prefer a cooler smoothie, you can add ice and blend again until it's completely crushed.

5. **Serve:** Pour the smoothie into a glass and serve immediately.

This green smoothie is packed with vitamins, minerals, fiber, and antioxidants. Spinach provides iron and folate, the apple and banana add natural sweetness and fiber, while ginger offers anti-inflammatory properties. Chia seeds add omega-3s and further fiber, making it a balanced and nutritious meal or snack.

Acai Bowl with Mixed Berries and Chia Seeds

Ingredients:

- 2 tablespoons of Acai powder or 1 packet of frozen Acai pulp

- 1 ripe banana

- 1/2 cup of mixed berries (such as strawberries, raspberries, blueberries)

- 1 cup of almond milk or other plant-based milk

- 1 tablespoon of chia seeds

- 1 tablespoon of honey or maple syrup (optional)

- Toppings: additional berries, unsweetened granola, shredded coconut

Nutritional Values (per serving):

- Calories: about 300-350 kcal

- Protein: 5-7 g

- Fats: 10-15 g

- Carbohydrates: 50-60 g

- Fiber: 10-12 g

- Sugars: 20-25 g

Preparation:

1. **Prepare the Ingredients:** Peel the banana and prepare the berries. If using frozen Acai, let it thaw for a few minutes to ease blending.

2. **Blend the Base:** Put the Acai powder (or thawed pulp), banana, mixed berries, almond milk, and chia seeds in a blender. Add the sweetener if desired. Blend until smooth and creamy.

3. **Assemble the Bowl:** Pour the mixture into a bowl.

4. **Add the Toppings:** Top the mixture with fresh berries, a handful of granola, and some shredded coconut for a crunchy and nutritious touch.

5. **Serve:** Enjoy your Acai bowl immediately to make the most of its freshness and creaminess.

This Acai bowl is an excellent option for breakfast or as an energizing snack. Acai is known for its antioxidant properties, while chia seeds provide omega-3s and fiber. The berries add vitamins and natural sweetness, making this dish not only healthy but also delicious.

Chicken Breast with Curry and Coconut Milk

Ingredients:

- 4 chicken breasts (about 150-200 g each)

- 1 can of coconut milk (about 400 ml)

- 2 tablespoons of curry paste (red or green, depending on preference)

- 1 medium onion, chopped

- 2 cloves of garlic, minced

- 1 piece of fresh ginger (about 2 cm), grated

- 1 tablespoon of extra virgin olive oil

- Salt and black pepper, to taste

- Fresh cilantro for garnish (optional)

Nutritional Values (per serving):

- Calories: about 350-400 kcal

- Protein: 25-30 g

- Fats: 20-25 g

- Carbohydrates: 8-10 g

- Fiber: 1-2 g

- Sugars: 3-4 g

Preparation:

1. **Prepare the Chicken:** Cut the chicken breasts into medium pieces. Season them lightly with salt and pepper.

2. **Sauté the Spices:** In a large skillet, heat the olive oil over medium heat. Add the chopped onion, garlic, and ginger. Cook until the onion is translucent.

3. **Add the Curry:** Add the curry paste to the skillet and mix well with the onions, garlic, and ginger. Cook for a minute to develop the flavors.

4. **Cook the Chicken:** Add the chicken pieces to the skillet and mix them with the spices to coat evenly. Cook for about 5-7 minutes or until the chicken starts to brown.

5. **Add the Coconut Milk:** Pour the coconut milk into the skillet, mixing well with the chicken and spices. Bring to a boil, then reduce the heat and simmer for 10-15 minutes, until the chicken is cooked through and the sauce has slightly thickened.

6. **Garnish and Serve:** Garnish the dish with chopped fresh cilantro, if desired. Serve the curry chicken with basmati rice or naan bread for a complete meal.

This dish combines the richness of coconut milk with the intense flavors of curry, creating a flavorful yet simple to prepare dish. The chicken provides a good source of protein, while the coconut milk adds creaminess and an exotic touch.

Chickpea Hummus with Smoked Paprika and Olive Oil

Ingredients:

- 1 can of chickpeas (about 400 g), drained and rinsed

- 2 tablespoons of tahini (sesame paste)

- 1 clove of garlic, minced

- The juice of 1 lemon

- 2 tablespoons of extra virgin olive oil, plus a bit more for garnish

- 1/2 teaspoon of smoked paprika

- Salt and black pepper, to taste

- Water or chickpea cooking water, if necessary

- For garnish: chopped parsley, sesame seeds, a pinch of paprika

Nutritional Values (per serving):

- Calories: about 150-200 kcal

- Protein: 6-8 g

- Fats: 8-10 g

- Carbohydrates: 15-20 g

- Fiber: 4-5 g

- Sugars: 2-3 g

Preparation:

1. **Prepare the Chickpeas:** Drain and rinse the chickpeas. For a creamier hummus, you can remove the skins that cover the chickpeas.

2. **Blend the Ingredients:** In a blender or food processor, combine the chickpeas, tahini, garlic, lemon juice, olive oil, smoked paprika, salt, and pepper. Blend until smooth and creamy. If the hummus is too thick, add a little water or chickpea cooking water to reach the desired consistency.

3. **Taste and Adjust:** Taste the hummus and adjust for salt, pepper, or lemon if necessary.

4. **Serve:** Transfer the hummus to a bowl. Create a small well in the center and drizzle with extra virgin olive oil. Sprinkle with chopped parsley, sesame seeds, and a pinch of paprika for garnish.

5. **Storage:** The hummus can be stored in the refrigerator in an airtight container for 3-4 days.

Chickpea hummus is an excellent source of plant-based protein and fiber. The addition of tahini provides healthy fats, while the smoked paprika adds a unique flavor touch. It's perfect as an appetizer, spread on toasted bread, or as a dip for raw vegetables.

Vegetarian Risotto with Zucchini and Basil

Ingredients:

- 1 cup of Arborio or Carnaroli rice (for risotto)

- 2 medium zucchinis, diced

- 1 small onion, finely chopped

- 2 cloves of garlic, minced

- 1 liter of vegetable broth

- 1/2 cup of dry white wine

- 2 tablespoons of extra virgin olive oil

- 1/4 cup of grated Parmesan cheese (optional for vegan version)

- A bunch of fresh basil, chopped

- Salt and black pepper, to taste

Nutritional Values (per serving):

- Calories: about 300-350 kcal

- Protein: 8-10 g

- Fats: 10-12 g

- Carbohydrates: 45-50 g

- Fiber: 2-3 g

- Sugars: 3-4 g

Preparation:

1. **Prepare the Broth:** Bring the vegetable broth to a boil and keep it warm over low heat.

2. **Sauté Onion and Garlic:** In a large pot, heat the olive oil and sauté the chopped onion until transparent. Add the garlic and cook for another minute.

3. **Add the Zucchini:** Put the diced zucchini in the pot and cook for about 3-4 minutes, until they start to soften.

4. **Toast the Rice:** Add the rice and toast for 1-2 minutes, stirring constantly.

5. **Deglaze with Wine:** Pour in the white wine and let it evaporate, stirring continuously.

6. **Cook the Risotto:** Begin adding the hot broth, one ladle at a time, waiting for the rice to almost completely absorb the liquid before adding the next. Continue this process for about 18-20 minutes, until the rice is al dente.

7. **Cream the Risotto:** Remove the pot from the heat and add the Parmesan cheese and fresh basil. Mix well until the risotto becomes creamy.

8. **Season:** Adjust salt and pepper to your taste.

9. **Serve:** Serve the risotto warm, garnished with additional fresh basil if desired.

This vegetarian risotto offers a great combination of complex carbohydrates, fiber, and proteins (especially if you add the Parmesan), as well as being rich in flavor thanks to the freshness of the zucchini and basil.

Whole Wheat Tortillas with Grilled Vegetable Filling

Ingredients:

- 4 whole wheat tortillas

- 1 zucchini, thinly sliced

- 1 red bell pepper, cut into strips

- 1 red onion, sliced

- 1 clove of garlic, minced

- 1 avocado, sliced

- 1 tomato, sliced

- 2 tablespoons of extra virgin olive oil

- Salt and black pepper, to taste

- Juice of 1 lime

- Chopped fresh cilantro (optional)

Nutritional Values (per serving):

- Calories: about 200-250 kcal

- Protein: 6-8 g

- Fats: 10-12 g (primarily monounsaturated fats from avocado)

- Carbohydrates: 30-35 g

- Fiber: 5-7 g

- Sugars: 4-6 g

Preparation:

1. **Grill the Vegetables:** Preheat a grill or grill pan over medium-high heat. Lightly coat the zucchini slices, bell pepper, and onion with one tablespoon of olive oil, salt, and pepper. Grill the vegetables for about 3-4 minutes per side, until they are tender and slightly charred.

2. **Prepare the Avocado:** In a bowl, mash the avocado with lime juice, minced garlic, salt, and pepper. Mix until you get a creamy consistency.

3. **Warm the Tortillas:** Warm the tortillas in a pan for about 30 seconds on each side, until they are soft and warm.

4. **Assemble the Tortillas:** Spread a portion of the mashed avocado on each tortilla. Add the grilled vegetables and tomato slices on top.

5. **Add Cilantro:** Sprinkle with chopped fresh cilantro, if desired.

6. **Serve:** Roll up the tortillas and serve immediately.

This recipe offers a light yet satisfying meal, rich in fiber and essential nutrients. The addition of avocado provides healthy fats, while the grilled vegetables add flavor and texture. The whole wheat tortillas increase the fiber content, making this meal a balanced and nutritious choice.

Avocado and Cocoa Mousse with Toasted Hazelnuts

Ingredients:

- 2 ripe avocados, peeled and pitted

- 1/4 cup of unsweetened cocoa powder

- 1/4 cup of honey or maple syrup (for a vegan version)

- 1/2 teaspoon of vanilla extract

- A pinch of salt

- 1/4 cup of almond milk or other plant-based milk

- 1/4 cup of hazelnuts, toasted and coarsely chopped

Nutritional Values (per serving):

- Calories: about 250-300 kcal

- Protein: 4-5 g

- Fats: 15-20 g (primarily monounsaturated and polyunsaturated fats from avocado)

- Carbohydrates: 25-30 g

- Fiber: 7-9 g

- Sugars: 12-15 g

Preparation:

1. **Blend the Ingredients:** Place the avocado, cocoa powder, honey or maple syrup, vanilla extract, salt, and almond milk in a blender or food processor. Blend until you achieve a smooth and creamy mixture. If necessary, add a little more milk to reach the desired consistency.

2. **Toast the Hazelnuts:** Preheat the oven to 180°C (350°F). Spread the hazelnuts on a baking sheet and toast them for 5-10 minutes, until they become lightly golden. Let them cool, then chop them coarsely.

3. **Assemble the Mousse:** Pour the mousse into individual bowls.

4. **Add the Hazelnuts:** Sprinkle the mousse with the chopped toasted hazelnuts.

5. **Chill:** Refrigerate the mousse for at least 1 hour before serving. This allows the mousse to firm up and fully develop its flavors.

6. **Serve:** Serve the mousse cold as a dessert or as a rich and nutritious snack.

This avocado and cocoa mousse is a rich and creamy dessert, yet surprisingly healthy. The avocado provides good fats and a creamy texture, while the cocoa adds a rich antioxidant flavor. The toasted hazelnuts add a delightful crunchy contrast.

Conclusion: Begin Your Journey Toward a Transformed Life

As we approach the end of our journey through the pages of "The Anti-Inflammatory Diet: Your Ally for Health," it's time to reflect not just on what we've learned but also on the power each of us holds to transform our lives. This book is not merely a guide but a beginning, a first step on a path that promises not only health but renewed well-being and vitality.

Yes, the journey toward an anti-inflammatory existence may seem daunting at first. Changing long-established habits, adopting new ways of eating, incorporating exercise into your daily routine, and managing stress in healthy ways requires commitment and determination. However, remember that every great journey begins with a single step. And you have already taken that step by starting to read these pages.

Imagine a life where the food you consume is no longer an enemy but a friend that nourishes, heals, and invigorates. A life where physical activity is not a burdensome task but a joyful opportunity to celebrate what your body can do. A life where stress doesn't dominate but is managed with grace and understanding through mindfulness and relaxation practices. This is the potential of what awaits you.

The anti-inflammatory journey is not just a path to symptom reduction or improved physical health. It's a road to a better understanding of yourself, to a deeper connection with the food you eat, the way you move your body, and the techniques you use to calm your mind. It's a journey that unites body, mind, and spirit in harmony that resonates in every aspect of your life.

As you continue on this path, there will inevitably be obstacles and challenges. But remember, each challenge is an opportunity to grow, to learn something new about yourself and the world around you. Don't be discouraged when you encounter an obstacle; rather, embrace it as a sign that you're making progress, that you're pushing your limits and discovering your true strength.

You are not alone on this journey. There are communities, both online and offline, filled with individuals who, like you, have chosen to embrace this lifestyle. These communities can offer support, advice, and inspiration. Share your story, listen to others', and together, grow.

In conclusion, these pages do not mark the end but rather a new beginning. A beginning of a journey that is as unique as you are. Take what you've learned, adapt it to your personal needs and circumstances, and look forward to the future with excitement. A future where each day brings you closer to the healthiest, happiest, and most fulfilled version of yourself.

Begin this journey with hope in your heart, with science and wisdom as your allies, and with the conviction that the anti-inflammatory path is more than a diet or a regimen – it's a new way of living fully, consciously, and joyously. Safe travels on your journey to your renewed self.

If this book has positively impacted you and been helpful, I would be grateful if you could take a moment to share your thoughts with a brief review on Amazon.

Thank you,

Giuliano Monti

Made in the USA
Monee, IL
18 October 2024

68201206R00089